Knee Surgery - Reconstruction and Replacement

Edited by João Bosco Sales Nogueira, José Alberto Dias Leite, Leonardo Heráclio Do Carmo Araújo and Marcelo Cortez Bezerra

Published in London, United Kingdom

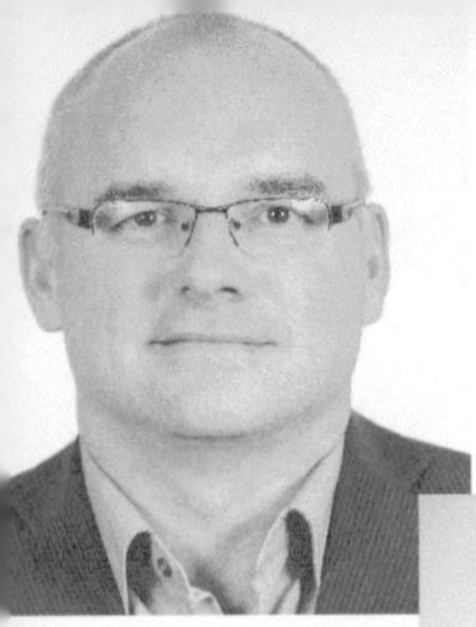
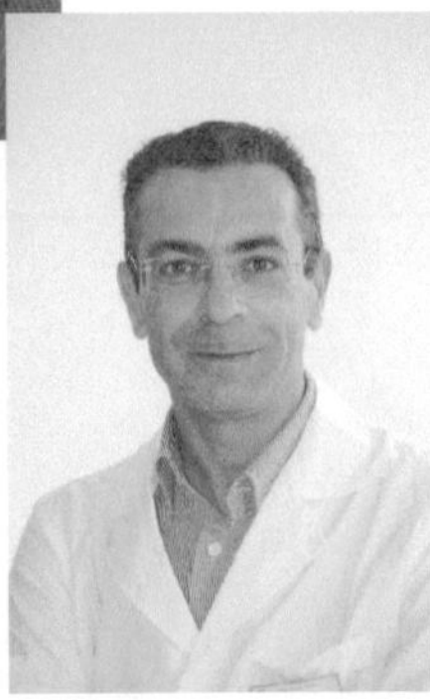
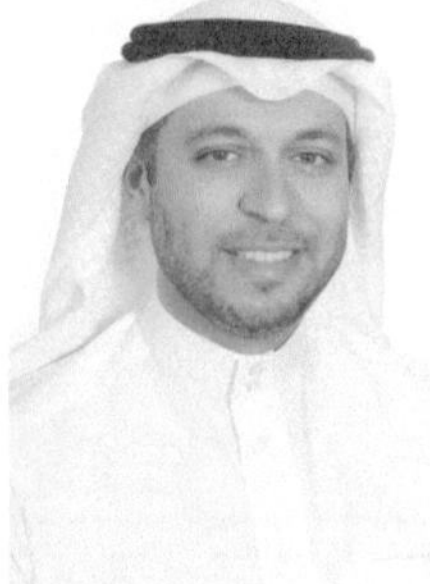
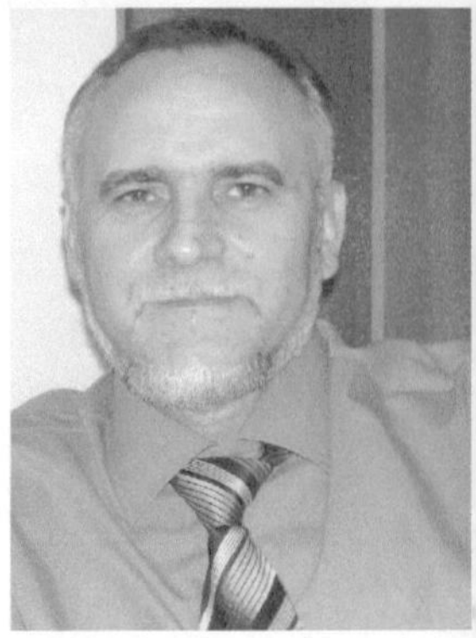
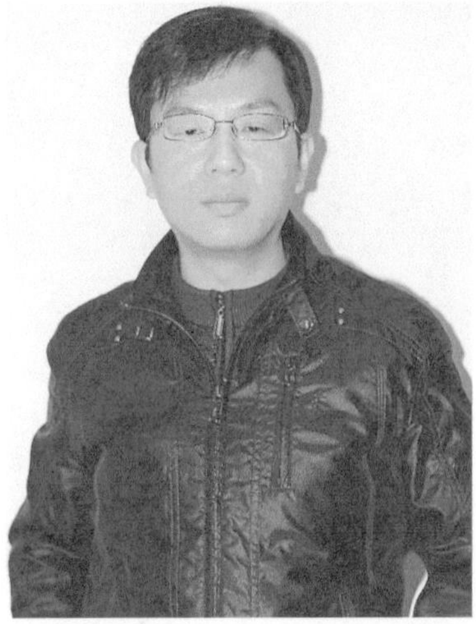
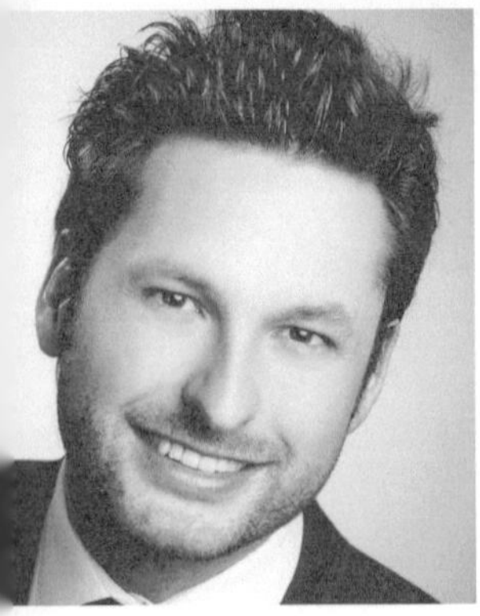
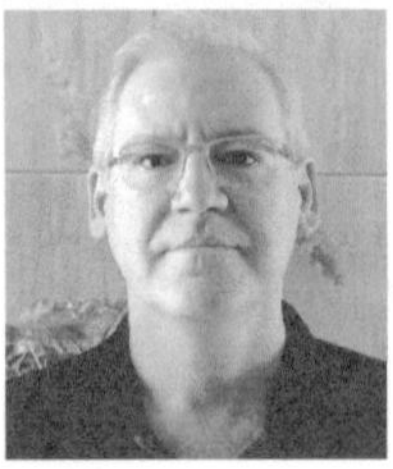

IntechOpen

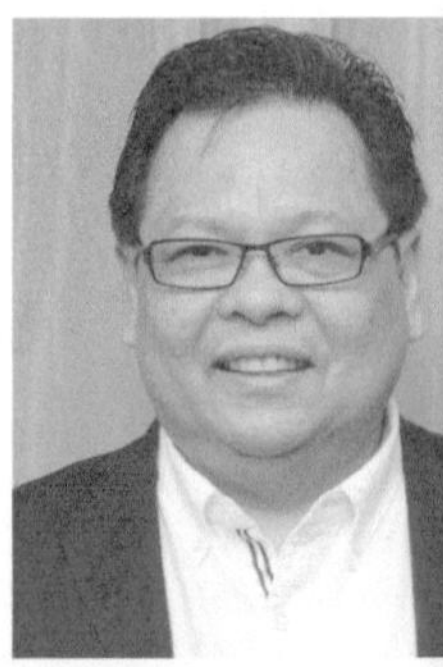
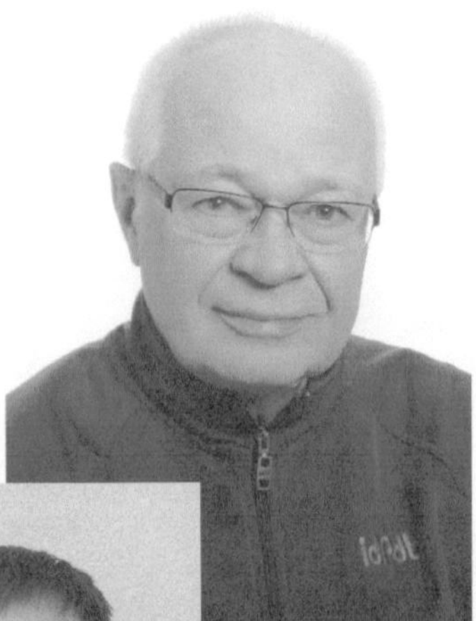
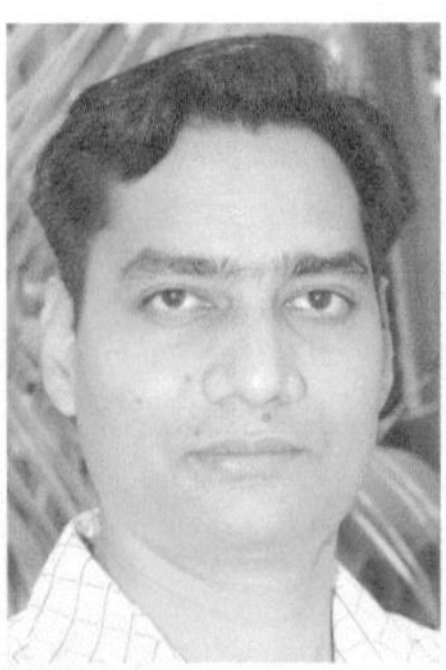
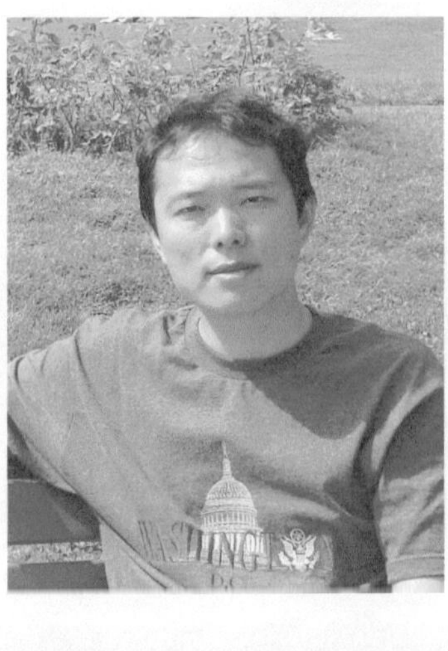
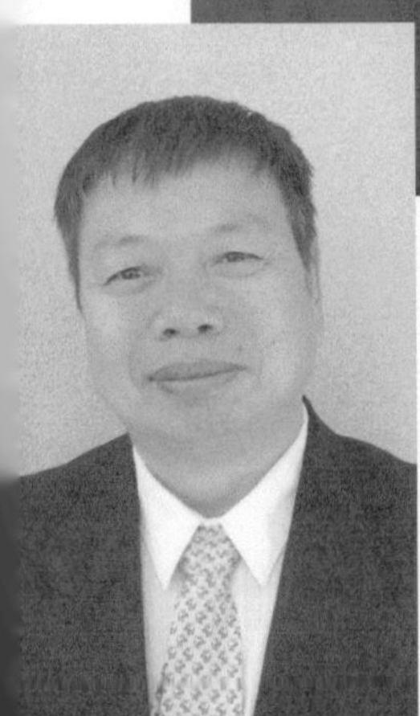
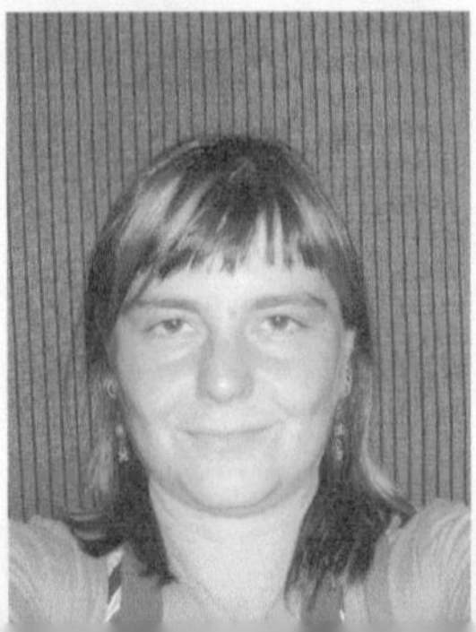

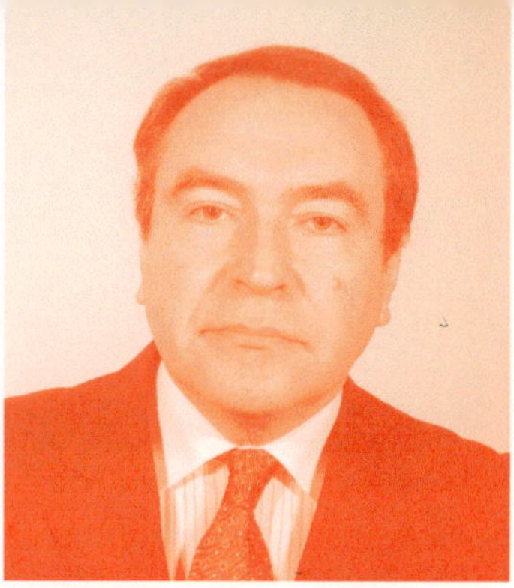
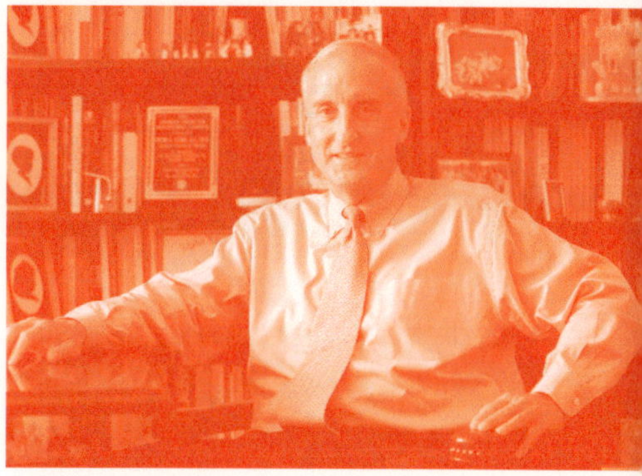
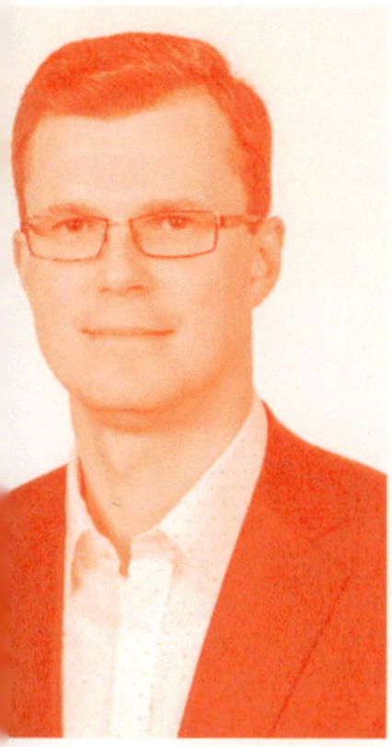
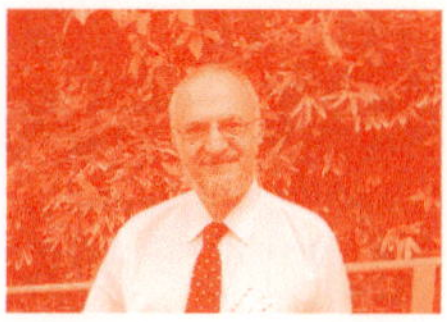
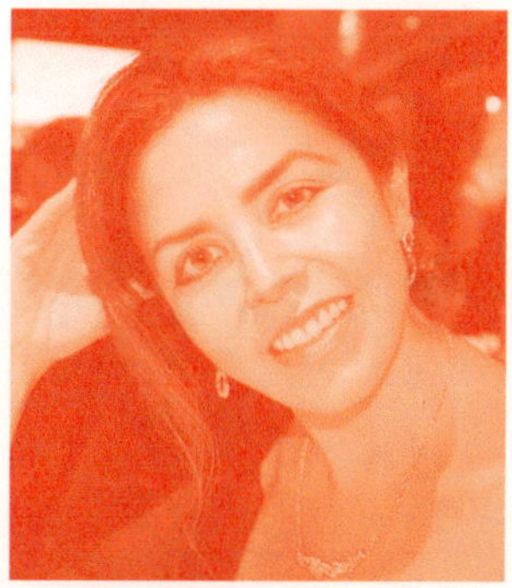

Supporting open minds since 2005

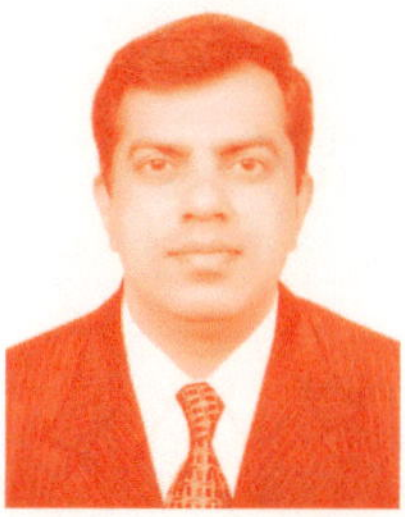
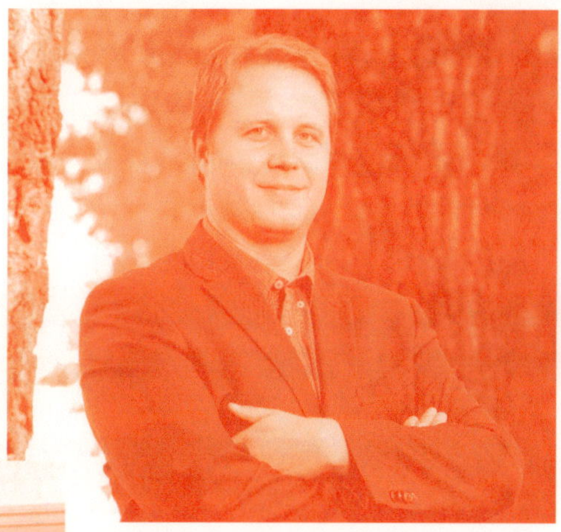
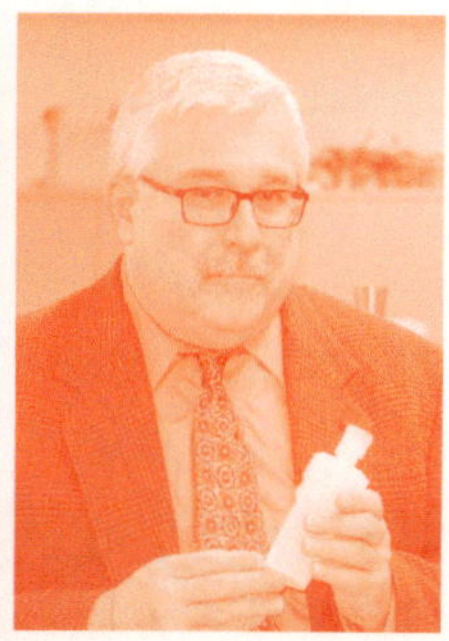
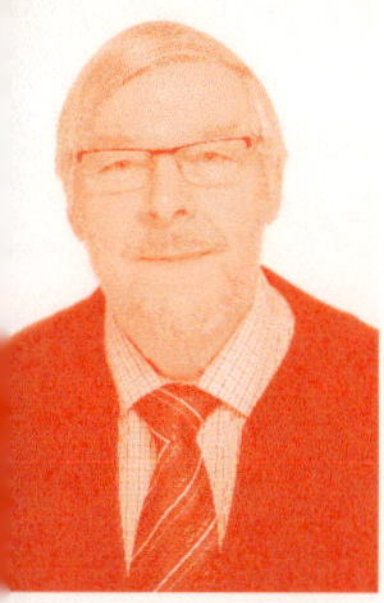
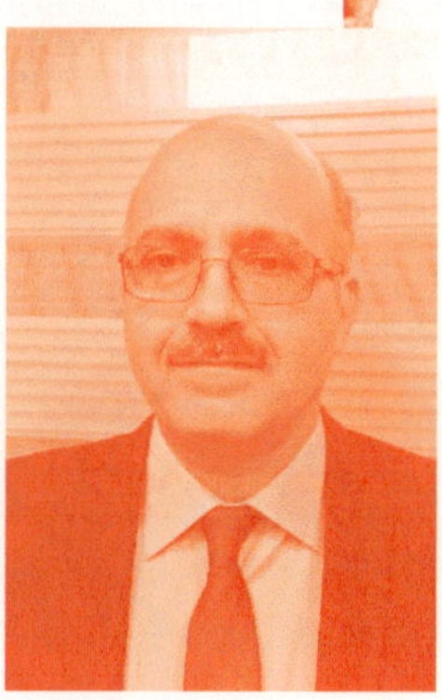
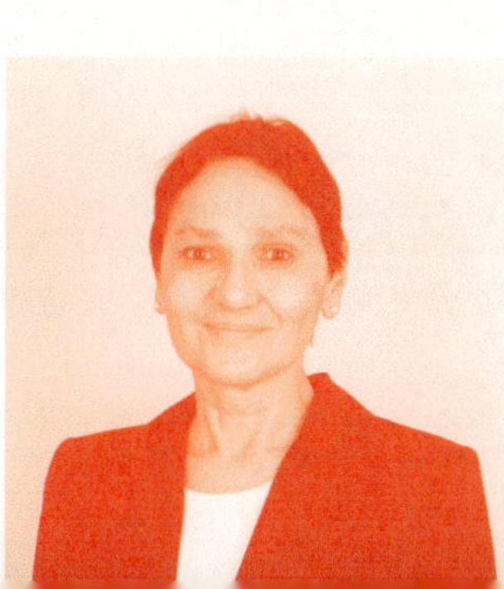
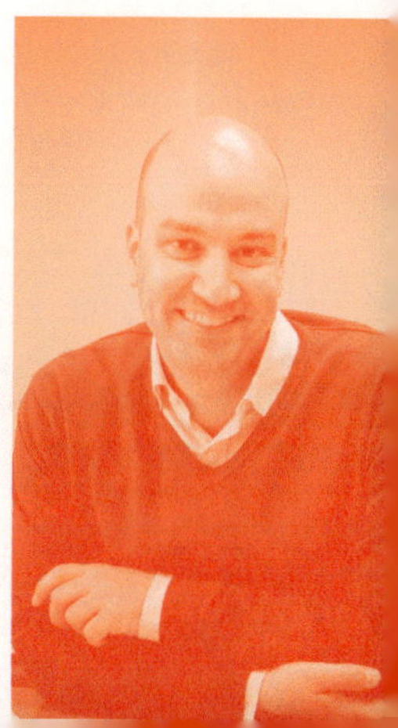

Knee Surgery - Reconstruction and Replacement
http://dx.doi.org/10.5772/intechopen.83631
Edited by João Bosco Sales Nogueira, José Alberto Dias Leite, Leonardo Heráclio Do Carmo Araújo and Marcelo Cortez Bezerra

Contributors
Wangdo Kim, Guillem Navarro, Oscar Ares, Ignacio Moya, Roberto Seijas, Pilar Camacho, Alonso Zumbado, Manuel Llusa, Andreu Combalia, Andrea Sallent, Tahsin Gurpinar, Gabriel Stan, Alisina Shahi, Vishavpreet Singh, Galen Berdis, Akshay Goel, Ali Oliashirazi, Kavin Khatri, Deepak Bansal, Karan Rajpal, Melvin George, Muhammet Salih Ayas, Muhammet Kalkışım, Ahmet Köse, Orkun Gül

First published in London, United Kingdom, 2020 by IntechOpen
IntechOpen is the global imprint of INTECHOPEN LIMITED, registered in England and Wales, registration number: 11086078, 7th floor, 10 Lower Thames Street, London, EC3R 6AF, United Kingdom
Printed in Croatia

British Library Cataloguing-in-Publication Data
A catalogue record for this book is available from the British Library

Additional hard and PDF copies can be obtained from orders@intechopen.com

Knee Surgery - Reconstruction and Replacement
Edited by João Bosco Sales Nogueira, José Alberto Dias Leite, Leonardo Heráclio Do Carmo Araújo and Marcelo Cortez Bezerra
p. cm.
Print ISBN 978-1-83880-530-2
Online ISBN 978-1-83880-531-9
eBook (PDF) ISBN 978-1-78985-062-8

For EU product safety concerns:
IN TECH d.o.o., Prolaz Marije Krucifikse Kozulić 3, 51000 Rijeka, Croatia, info@intechopen.com or visit our website at intechopen.com.

Meet the editors

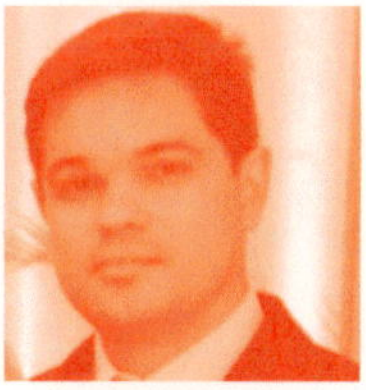

João Bosco Sales Nogueira received his MD, MsC, and PhD candidate from the Universidade Federal do Ceara, Brazil. He is a coordinator of the Knee Surgery Internship of Santa Casa de Fortaleza/Centro do Joelho, a member of the International Society of Arthroscopy, Knee Surgery, and Orthopedic Sports Medicine (ISAKOS), a member of the Sociedade Brasileira de Cirurgia do Joelho (SBCJ), and a member of the Sociedade Brasileira de Ortopedia e Traumatologia (SBOT).

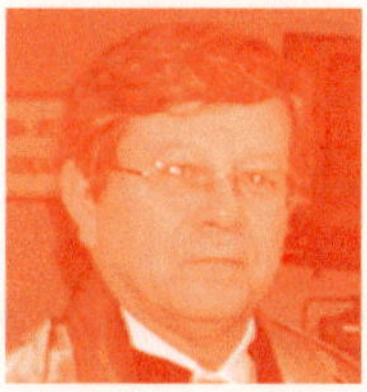

José Alberto Dias Leite graduated in Medicine from the Rio de Janeiro School of Medicine and Surgery. He has a master's degree and doctorate in Medicine from the Federal University of Rio de Janeiro and a degree in Teaching from the State University of Rio de Janeiro. He is currently a full professor at the Department of Surgery at the Federal University of Ceará, Head of the Orthopedics and Traumatology Service at the Walter Cantídio University Hospital at the Federal University of Ceará, Vice-Coordinator of the Postgraduate Program in Medical and Surgical Sciences, School of Medicine, Federal University of Ceará, and Professor of Orthopedics at UNICHRISTUS. He has experience in medicine, focusing on orthopedic surgery, especially osteoarticular stress.

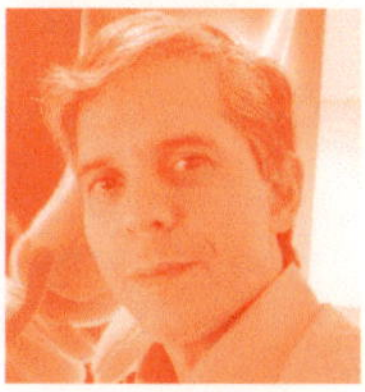

Dr. Leonardo Heráclio Do Carmo Araújo graduated from the Federal University of Ceara, Orthopedics and Knee Surgery at Campinas University (Unicamp) He did a fellowship on Knee Surgery at the Centre Hospitalier du Nord Isére, Lyon, France. He is currently a knee surgery preceptor at Santa Casa da Misericórdia de Fortaleza, a professor of Medical Practices at Ceara State University (UECE), and a member of the Brazilian Knee Surgery Society (SBCJ), ISAKOS.

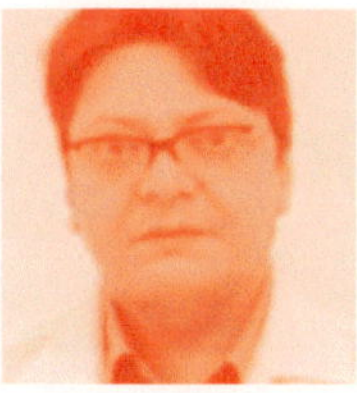

Dr. Marcelo Cortez Bezerra graduated in orthopedics and knee surgery at Santa Casa de Misericórdia of São Paulo. He obtained his master's degree in Surgery from the Federal University of Ceara. He is a medical school professor at Fortaleza University (Unifor), Chairman of Orthopedic Surgery at Santa Casa da Misericórdia de Fortaleza, and a member of the Brazilian Knee Surgery Society (SBCJ), ISAKOS.

Contents

Preface

Knee Surgery—Reconstruction and Replacement is an intriguing book that addresses the most common injuries noted in a knee surgeon's routine, from biomechanical aspects to special situations of ligament injuries and joint replacement surgeries. It is not a compendium, or a base book, but an update book, complementary to the life of the knee specialist.

João Bosco Sales Nogueira (Editor) and José Alberto Dias Leite (Co-editor)
Programa de Pós Graduação em Cirurgia da Faculdade de Medicina da Universidade Federal do Ceara. (Post Graduation Program of Medicine School of Federal University of Ceara, Brazil)

Leonardo Heráclio do Carmo Araújo (Co-editor)
Santa Casa de Fortaleza,
Brazil

Marcelo José Cortez Bezerra (Co-editor)
Santa Casa de Fortaleza,
Brazil
University of Fortaleza,
Brazil

Section 1

Biomechanics

Chapter 1

Tibial Femoral Tunnel for Isokinetic Graft Placement Based on a Tensegrity Model of a Knee

Wangdo Kim

Abstract

We characterize the concept of a "knee axis" and further the concept of "invariant." It is now generally recognized that one of the features of the tensegrity (*prestressable to the same configuration*) allows the knee tensegrity system to be in producing the knee instantaneous axis (KIA). We found that the line of the ground reaction force (GRF) vector is very close to the KIA. It aligns the knee joint with the GRF such that the reaction forces are torqueless. The reaction to the GRF will then be carried by the whole structures on the knee tensegrity instead. The use of knee tensegrity model introduces the new useful dimensions of sensitivity in foot loading to the knee axis alignment. We demonstrated a method to determine ideal placement of the tibial tunnel with respect to the KIA. Such placement in vivo has the potential to reliably produce an isokinetic graft without risk of impingement.

Keywords: knee tensegrity system, knee instantaneous axis, the haptic perceptual system, knee alignment

1. Introduction

The perceptual psychologist James J. Gibson regarded the senses as aggressively seeking mechanisms rather than mere passive receivers [1]. The active movement involves the concomitant operation of anatomical components, in which foot touches the ground and rotation of the joints are combined, together with voluntary contractions of the muscles. The total flux of stimulation involved in the so-called active movement is enormously complex, but lawful modes of combination occur. Presumably, the modes of combination of these inputs specify the difference between touching (active) and being touched (passive) [2].

To identify the haptic system's medium, Turvey focused on connective tissue and the conjunction of muscular, connective tissue net, and skeletal as the body's proper characterization [3]. Myers has also posed the medium as a body-wide responsive physiological network—the myofascial meridian [4]. Taking on "geometry" first, cell biologist Donald Ingber placed one final piece of the puzzle: to view the body's architecture in the light of "tensegrity" geometry [5]. "Tensegrity" was coined from the phrase "tension integrity" by the designer R. Buckminster Fuller (working from original structures developed by artist Kenneth Snelson) [6].

The principle of tensegrity describes precisely the relationship between the connective tissues, the muscles, and the skeleton. Weight applied to shank/thigh bones would cause it to slide off its knee joint if it were not for the tensional balances that hold it in place and control its pivoting [7]. The invariant feature of tensegrity structures encompasses those that stabilize themselves through a phenomenon known as prestressing. Architects call this type of prestressed structural network, composed of opposing tension and compression elements that self-stabilizes its shape through the establishment of a mechanical force balance, a tensegrity structure. Biotensegrity is a term introduced by Dr. Stephen Levin and denotes the application of tensegrity's principles to biological structures [8].

Tensional forces naturally transmit themselves over the shortest distance between two points, so the elastic members of tensegrity structures are precisely positioned to best withstand applied stress. For this reason, tensegrity structures offer a maximum amount of strength for any given amount of material [4]. The invariant feature of a knee tensegrity system (specified by a given set of *external forces such as the ground reaction force* (*GRF*)) is a stable equilibrium if the structure returns to the originally given configuration after the application of arbitrarily small perturbations with respect to the KIA anywhere within the configuration [5] (**Figure 1**).

Consequently, estimating of the knee axis is one of the key topics for the "2010 ASME Grand Challenge Competition to Predict in Vivo Knee Loads" [11]. Knee functional axis information is referred to the knee instantaneous axis (KIA)

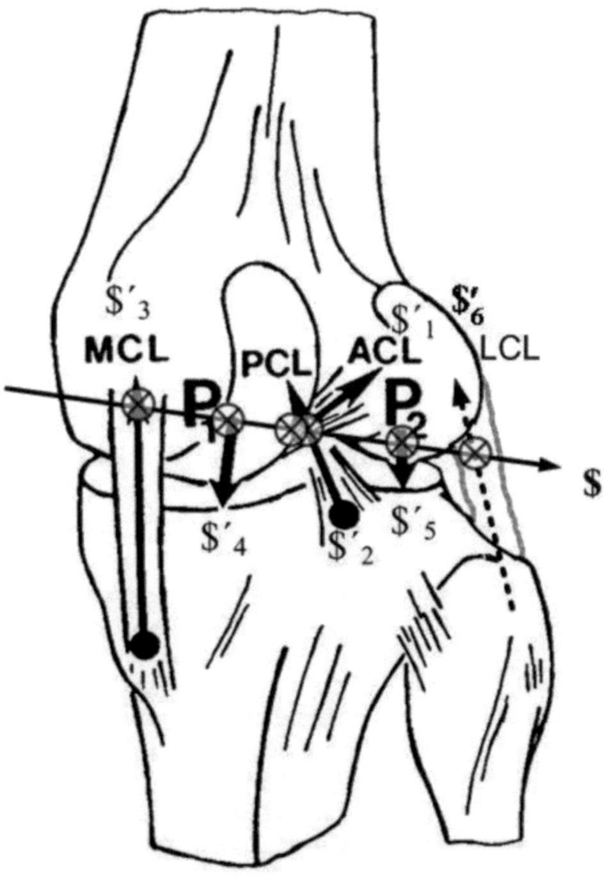

Figure 1.
The tensegrity structure of surrounding forces applied to the knee joint: a native system of the knee where six constraints $' are collectively reciprocal to the KIA $ indicated by ⊗ that the virtual coefficient should vanish is necessary, and sufficient conditions [9, 10], or the pair ($' and $) are in involution. The tensegrity's structure is characterized by the contact normal elements $'$_4$ and $'$_5$, while all the other elements are, continuous tension elements, showing specific configuration having torqueless connections.

[12–14]. In that case, the intersegmental force such as ligaments and contact forces are in pure tension/compression and are surrounding the KIA in such a way that those forces result in no (virtual) works [9, 10].

The objective of this study is to show how the knee tensegrity system manages the balance between tension and compression during locomotion by utilizing a unique combination of the KIA and GRF stimuli.

2. Materials and methods

The intra-articular structures of the tensegrity system of the knee include the muscles, the anterior cruciate ligament (ACL), posterior cruciate ligament (PCL), medial collateral ligament (MCL), and articular contact in the medial (P_1) and lateral (P_2) compartments (**Figure 1**) [15]. We have shown that six constraints are members of the "joint reaction subspace (JRS)" and are spatially oriented in such ways that by imposing an internal tension or "prestress" to reduce the play in the system, this ensures immediate mechanical responsiveness (i.e., that movement of one element is felt by all others) and reduces impact fatigue at the joint.

3. Results and discussion

We have measured the KIA through readily accessible benchmark data [11]. Also, we have measured the GRF on how the progression of the entire body over the limb uses the so-called rockers on foot. The issues of relating the reciprocal connection of the body framework to the movements of cutaneous kinesthesis [9, 10, 15, 16] (zoomed up the pan in **Figure 2**) enunciate that the body's haptic perceptual system registers the covariance of the KIA and GRF. The upward pressure on the surface of support on the ventral side of the foot provides, for every terrestrial animal, a continuous background of stimulation. It is covariant with the continuous input of the appropriate receptors of the articular motion in the knee joint already mentioned. Together they provide what the ordinary person calls the "sense of support."

A unique combination of invariants, such as the KIA and GRF, a *compound* invariant, is just another invariant. It is a unit, and the components do not have to be combined or associated. Only if percepts were combinations of sensations would they have to be associated. Otherwise, we can postulate that when the KIA and GRF are completely covariant when they *always* go together, they constitute a single "stimulus." If the knee tensegrity system is capable of extracting invariants from changing haptic stimuli, there is no reason why it should not extract invariants that seem to us highly complex. Therefore, the reaction torque caused by the foot-ground at the knee will be taken on partially by muscles surrounding the joint.

Perception is not based on the structure of force as it falls upon the plantar side of the foot, the erroneous theory of the passive, sense-datum theory, but on continuous modifications brought about by foot movement which cooperates with body posture to reveal its invariants—a surface of support. The pattern of a compound invariant may indicate the neural loops of an active perceptual system that includes the adjustments of the perceptual organs, our locomotor apparatus. We may suppose that the brain governs the orienting of the organs of perception so that the whole locomotor system of afferent/efferent loops resonates to the patterns of compound invariants [17]. Locomotion is controlled not by the brain, but

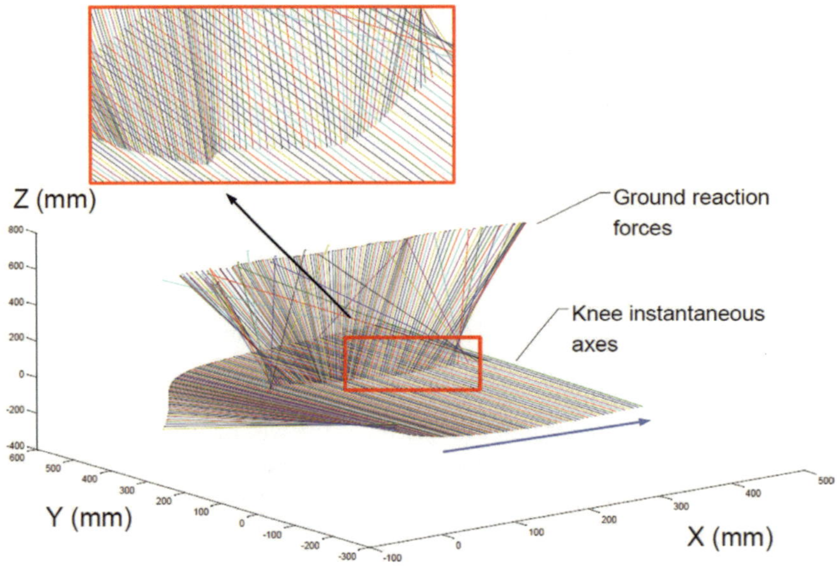

Figure 2.
A unique combination of the KIA and GRF invariant. When deformed by the shank to the ground via GRF, the strain is distributed over the whole structure, not localized in the area being deformed, i.e., the joint itself. A reaction torque is zero on the knee joint if the GRF line of action intersects the joint axis, or the configuration can exert a large force on the ground without overloading the knee joint. A considerable ground reaction force can be exerted on a foot when the vector nearly coincides with a reciprocal screw of joints. It is indicative of the "sense of support" being manifested based on the close correspondence of the vector of the ground reaction force at COP, and the IAK with fluctuations at the spatial scale of a millimeter (GRF-KIA coupling).

by information. We showed that the GRF might reciprocally be used to control locomotion.

We should choose surgical procedures that not only reconstruct the anatomy but also restore the articular kinesthesis, that is, the pickup of own movement [18–21]. In such an application, avoiding roof impingement during reconstruction of a torn ACL might find benefit in choosing a tunnel placement that can come near to a tensegrity model of a knee.

We found that the line of the ground reaction force (GRF) vector is very close to the KIA. It aligns the knee joint with the GRF such that the reaction forces are torqueless. The reaction to the GRF will then be carried by the whole structures on the knee tensegrity instead.

Conflicts of interest

The author declares no conflicts of interest.

Abbreviations

COP	center of pressure
GRF	ground reaction force
KIA	knee instantaneous axis

Author details

Wangdo Kim
Ingeniería Mecánica, Universidad de Ingenieria y Tecnologia - UTEC, Lima, Peru

*Address all correspondence to: mwdkim@gmail.com

References

[1] Gibson JJ. Observations on active touch. Psychological Review. 1962;**69**:477-491

[2] Gibson JJ. The Senses Considered as Perceptual Systems. Boston: Houghton; 1966

[3] Turvey MT, Fonseca ST. The medium of haptic perception: A tensegrity hypothesis. Journal of Motor Behavior. 2014;**46**(3):143-187

[4] Myers TW. Anatomy Trains: Myofascial Meridians for Manual and Movement Therapists. Edinburgh: Elsevier; 2014

[5] Ingber DE. The architecture of life. Scientific American. 1998;**278**(1):48-57

[6] Skelton RE, de Oliveira MC. Tensegrity Systems. Dordrecht/New York: Springer; 2009

[7] Swanson RL 2nd. Biotensegrity: A unifying theory of biological architecture with applications to osteopathic practice, education, and research—A review and analysis. The Journal of the American Osteopathic Association. 2013;**113**(1):34-52

[8] Hutson MA, Ellis RM. Textbook of Musculoskeletal Medicine. Oxford/New York: Oxford University Press; 2006

[9] Kim W, Veloso AP, Araújo D, Vleck V, João F. An informational framework to predict reaction of constraints using a reciprocally connected knee model. Computer Methods in Biomechanics and Biomedical Engineering. 2015;**18**(1):78-89

[10] Kim W, Veloso AP, Vleck VE, Andrade C, Kohles SS. The stationary configuration of the knee. Journal of the American Podiatric Medical Association. 2013;**103**(2):126-135

[11] Fregly BJ, Besier TF, Lloyd DG, Delp SL, Banks SA, Pandy MG, et al. Grand challenge competition to predict in vivo knee loads. Journal of Orthopaedic Research. 2012;**30**(4):503-513

[12] Kim W, Choi Y, Lee HG. The duality of knee functional axes and foot contact. Journal of Functional Morphology and Kinesiology. 2016;**1**(4):387

[13] Kim W, Choi Y, Lee H. Observations on the knee functional axis during active movements. SM Musculoskeletal Disorders. 2016;**1**(1):5

[14] Kim W, Kim YH, Veloso AP, Kohles SS. Tracking knee joint functional axes through Tikhonov filtering and Plűcker coordinates. Journal of Novel Physiotherapies. 1 Mar 2013; Suppl **4**(1):11732

[15] Kim W, Veloso A, Tan J, Andrade C. A reciprocal connection at knee joint. In: ASME 2010 Summer Bioengineering Conference; Naples, FL; 2010

[16] Kim W, Kohles SS. A reciprocal connection factor for assessing knee-joint function. Computer Methods in Biomechanics and Biomedical Engineering. 2011;**15**(9):911-917

[17] Gibson JJ. The visual perception of objective motion and subjective movement. Psychological Review. 1954;**61**(5):304-314

[18] Adrian CP, Haussler KK, Kawcak C, Reiser RF, Riegger-Krugh C, Palmer RH, et al. The role of muscle activation in cruciate disease. Veterinary Surgery. 2013;**42**(7):765-773

[19] Jerosch J, Prymka M. Knee joint proprioception in normal volunteers and patients with anterior cruciate ligament tears, taking special account of the effect of a knee bandage. Archives of Orthopaedic and Trauma Surgery. 1996;**115**(3-4):162-166

[20] Jerosch J, Prymka M. Knee joint proprioception in patients with posttraumatic recurrent patella dislocation. Knee Surgery, Sports Traumatology, Arthroscopy. 1996;**4**(1):14-18

[21] Jerosch J, Prymka M. Proprioception and joint stability. Knee Surgery, Sports Traumatology, Arthroscopy. 1996;**4**(3):171-179

Section 2

Ligament Injuries

Chapter 2

Ski Lesions Around the Knee: A Literature Review

Guillem Navarro Escarp, Oscar Ares Rodriguez, Ignacio Moya Molinas, Pilar Camacho Carrasco, Alonso Zumbado Dijeres, Roberto Seijas Vazquez, Andrea Sallent, Manuel Llusa Pérez and Andreu Combalia Aleu

Abstract

Ski is a popular sports practiced worldwide although it is considered a high-risk sports with high incidence of injuries. A common place for injuries is the knee, with a wide range from knee sprains to complex ligamentous injuries to fractures. In this chapter, we made a search in PubMed using the words "knee" and "ski." Later, we selected those articles according to the inclusion criteria. When reviewing the literature, we found that the most common place for a ski-related injury is the knee, with knee sprains and ACL lesions being the most common diagnosis in the latter years with a decreasing incidence of tibia fractures. We could also analyze the risk factors different authors have found, for professional athletes and for recreational skiers. In conclusion, the ACL lesion in the skier presents a high incidence, which suggests an effort should be made to prevent it.

Keywords: knee, ski, ACL, ligament, MCL

1. Introduction

Alpine skiing is a very popular sports with an increasing number of participants worldwide although being considered a high-risk sports with a high incidence of injuries in its participants. It is a sports with a great diversity in the profile and level of people practicing it, from amateur skiers to professional athletes with a high number of hours of exposure to injury risk.

Among the most frequent injuries, there are those affecting the knee joint, with a wide specter of severity: from mild sprains or contusions to serious multiligamentary injuries or complex fractures.

The aim of this study is to perform a literature review to assess the more common injuries in alpine skiing, see if there is a change in recent years due to new equipment and attitudes, look for its risk factors, and analyze possible preventive measures to reduce the risk of serious injuries.

2. Epidemiology

Alpine skiing is the most popular winter sports [1] worldwide. Only in the United States, more than 18 million people 5 years old or older participated in alpine skiing or snowboarding at least in one occasion in the 2011–2012 season [2], and there are about 200 million skiers worldwide [3]. Even more this popularity seems to be increasing all around the world.

Professional skiing is also a popular sports, with 3625 ski races arranged by the International Ski Federation (FIS) in the 2007–2008 season, of those 74 were Alpine Ski World Cup races in which up to 443 athletes participated [4]. Ski racing comprises diverse disciplines from aggressive-turning and highly technical demands like slalom to high speed with big jumps with almost no protective wear like downhill. Besides, alpine ski racing is a popular TV sports, with up to 250 million of TV spectators in 2009 according to FIS data.

It is a well-known fact that skiing is a sports with a high incidence of injuries, some estimate about 2.5–3 injuries per 1000 skier days in amateur practice [3], with head trauma and injuries around the knee being the most frequently reported. Knowing this data one can simply imagine the huge sanitary, social, and economic burden that skier injuries suppose in our societies.

3. Material and methods

A literature search was made using the PubMed database. We used keywords as ski and knee in order to maximize the number of results. In this first search, we obtained 285 results. We decided to include articles from 1995 to 2018 to be able to compare data published before many technological innovations were introduced with more recent data; this limited the number of articles to 211. All titles and abstracts were analyzed to identify the articles of interest: those investigating about the incidence, types, and risk factors for knee injuries during the practice of alpine skiing in adult population, either amateur or professional.

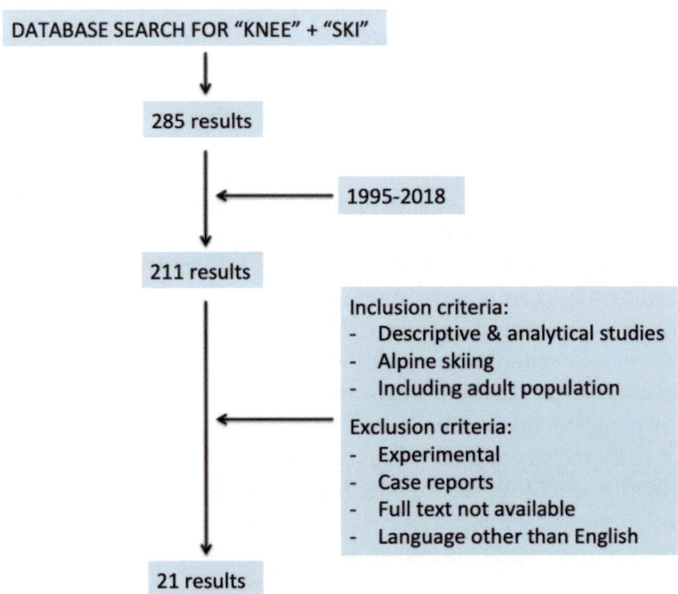

Figure 1.
Chart showing the selection process of our study.

Descriptive and analytical studies were included, and some reviews were taken into account for its particular interest and value. Experimental and laboratory studies were excluded, as well as case reports. We had to discard all articles not written in English and those whose complete text was not possible to obtain for any reason. All the process with its phases is detailed in **Figure 1**.

Given the reduced number of studies with high-quality evidence in knee injuries in alpine skiing, it was deemed that the best methodology was to do a narrative review.

4. Results

After applying the process explained in the previous point, we had 21 results, 18 original articles, and 3 reviews.

When analyzing all the studies, the first thing that stands out is the big variability between them. We could find studies referring to professional athletes and others to general amateur skiers. We could also find studies done in high-level trauma centers and others done in small ski resort clinics without a physician, with great differences in the diagnostics and clinical information reported. Moreover, the studies' designs also presented a great variability.

4.1 Athlete skiers

Referring to the alpine ski racers' population, Stenroos and Handolin [1] reported no differences in the absolute injury rate in men compared to women, although the mean age of their study is 14 years old, which in our opinion can produce some bias. The most common injury mechanism was the fall down on the same level, with 56% of injuries taking place on giant slalom runs (characterized by higher speed runs) and 31% on slalom runs. About 74% of injuries in this study group required hospitalization. Knee injuries represented the 34.4% of all injuries: 81% were ligamentous injuries being 47% of them anterior cruciate ligament (ACL) injuries (which means the ACL injuries were the 13% of the total). Ligamentous knee injuries were more common in women than in men; in the ACL group, 75% of injured skiers were women. Recovery after an ACL injury took a mean time of 175 days (range 150–180 days) without skiing, and all those patients reported mild or great discomfort in skiing 6 months after the injury. No knee fractures were reported; but 26% of injuries were leg (tibia and fibula) fractures, a surprising high rate when comparing to literature, probably due to the relative young age of this study population.

Similar results were reported by Schmitt et al. [5] in a study in athletes in the Swiss national ski teams. A knee injury rate of 35% was reported, with no differences between men and women; 71% were ACL injuries, of which 26% were isolated ACL injuries and 44% presented an associated injury of a collateral ligament and/or menisci. Their conclusion is that ACL is the most frequent knee injury in competitive alpine skiing. In their objective to describe risk factors for ACL injury, they report a higher risk in slalom runs (with more aggressive and technical turns but at lower speeds) and in athletes with better FIS score and rank, highlighting a higher prevalence of ACL ruptures in the top 30 World Cup skiers. Finally, body mass index, weight, and fitness status (assessed with a specific fitness test: Swiss Ski Power Test) did not correlate with ACL injury risk.

In two successive studies, Flørenes et al. [4] and Bere et al. [6] investigated the sex differences in risk injury in World Cup skiers, first for two seasons [4] and then for six seasons [6]. They report a mean absolute injury rate of 36.2 injuries/100 athletes/season with a higher relative injury rate in men (11.3 injuries/1000 runs) than in women (7.1 injuries/1000 runs). Of this 82.3% were time-loss injuries, with 43% being reported as severe (absence from skiing >28 days) and 31% moderate (absence 8–28 days). 45.5% of the injuries took place during the World Cup races. Knee injuries represented the 38% and lower leg and Achilles tendon injuries the 9%. In ACL injuries, there were no sex differences (5.4 ACL injuries/100 athletes/ season in men vs. 5.5 in women).

When analyzing knee injuries, they reported that 83% were ligamentous injuries, of which 45% were ACL injuries (that makes the ACL the most common ligament injury), and only 4.4% were fractures. They report that 50% of knee injuries are classified as severe. The relative ACL injury rate was higher in downhill and supergiant races (high speed with softer turns) than in giant and slalom races; this result matches with Stenroos' study results [1].

In [7, 8], Jordan et al. made a review in which they report literature finding that only 55% of alpine skiing athletes are able to return to their preinjury level after an ACL rupture. They also support the result we have found that in this group of skiers there is no sex difference in ACL injury rates.

4.2 Amateur skiers

Referring to amateur skiers, Patrick et al. [2] made a study comparing injury epidemiology in skiers between the 1996 and 2013 seasons. In both years, the knee was the most commonly injured body part (28%). An interesting fact they report is that helmet use augmented from only 6 to 84%, which means that although there is an increasing effort to make skiing a safer sports this has had no impact on the amount of knee injuries. They also report and increase in injuries among people older than 45 years. This results match with the published by Stenroos et al. [1] when they report an injury risk of 1 injury/10,000 ski lifts or in their calculation 1.97 injuries/1000 skier days in amateur people. Knee lesions were the 28.5% of the total, almost half of them being suspected as moderate or severe injuries. A major limitation in this study, which is also present in similar ones, is the lack of precise diagnostics, as data is collected by rescuers and/or in small ski resort clinics.

Continuing with the epidemiology review, Girardi et al. [9] studied factors affecting injury severity using the Injury Severity Score (ISS). They found that being a man and being older than 60 years were risk factors for an increased ISS, while the ISS was lower in beginner skiers and during a snowfall. There is no information in this article about these risk factors relating to knee injury risk. In [10], Khalilifar et al. report a lower knee injury rate, of only 14%, but this rate being higher in women, a result also found in other studies [11–14].

In [15], Davidson and Laliotis, a 9-year survey (from 1983 to 1992) of injury patterns in alpine skiers, reported an increase in injury rate from 1.9 to 3 injuries/1000 skier days. Knee injuries were 35%, and what is more relevant is a 92% increase in the number of knee injuries during their study period.

A very similar study period is researched by Warme et al. in [16] reporting a stable injury rate of 3.7 injuries/1000 skier days and knee injuries being 34% of the total. The most relevant part is that they report an exact diagnostic information (30% of the total on injuries affected the knee ligaments): 18% the medial collateral ligament (MCL), 16.5% the ACL, and in 20% of knee sprains, both ligaments were affected. They report a significant increase in ACL injuries.

Coury et al. [17] compared the epidemiology of skiing injuries in a ski resort clinic between 1995 and 2000 and the 2009/2010 seasons. Their results show also the knee injury as the most frequent (43%). Knee ligament sprain or strain was diagnosed in 25% on injured people, 10% with torn cruciate ligament, and 6% with what they call "internal derangement of the knee" (probably, a torn meniscus was to be diagnosed in this group of patients). Skiing injuries were more common in intermediate- or advanced-level skiers, but beginner skiers were the ones most at risk for knee injuries. They report only 3.2% on tibia and fibula fractures, and only 3.6% of ankle injuries in skiers, while snowboarders present up to 13% of ankle injuries. This difference may be explained by the use of hard-shell boots in ski.

A recent interesting study [18] discusses about injuries from 2001 to 2006 in a level 1 trauma center, which probably means a loss of minor injuries but on the other hand can inform about the most severe ones. They report a 52.3% of lower extremity injuries, the majority classified as soft tissue knee injuries but with a 2% of knee dislocation, 26% of tibia fractures (ankle not included), and 15.7% of femur fractures. The mean hospitalization rate was of 3.36 days, and 13.9% of patients required a surgical intervention. In our opinion, the high rates of severe injuries, especially major bone fractures, are because of a selection bias due to the nature of the hospital where the study took place. Results published by Ekeland et al. [19] support our conclusion: injury rate of 1.27 injuries/1000 skier days with leg fractures being only 3.6% in adult population. In children these fractures made up to 12.6% of injuries. They conclude that while there was a huge reduction in leg fractures during the 1970s–1980s probably due to higher quality of boots, making them higher and hard-shelled, and bindings, this reduction was not observed in children to the same degree.

In the same direction point, the article by Castellani et al. [14] reported that fractures in skiers are more common in men and especially in younger patients (<15 years old). Knee injuries are the most common (28.3–31.3% of injuries), with knee fractures being between 2 and 5%. A result that is important to be highlighted is their finding of an increased risk in women for knee ligamentous injury: men presented 14–15% of ligamentous knee injuries and 36–41% in women. In their data, the hospitalization rate was of 26%, from which 62% underwent surgery; mean hospital stay was 10.5–12.8 days. Knee arthroscopy was realized in 1.9–6.3% of operations. These results can be biased by the fact that almost half of injured patients were referred to their home hospital for treatment of lesions; and as ligamentous injuries are not a surgical emergency, the probability of being referred to in the presence of such an injury grows when compared to a patient with a fracture.

4.2.1 Risk factors in amateur skiers

Some studies did an effort to clarify which risk factors play a role in knee injuries in alpine skiers. As commented before this is a more heterogeneous group with big differences with respect to ski racers, so risk factors may be completely different.

Sulheim et al. [20] reported that beginners (OR 2.7) and children younger than 13 years old (OR 1.32) were more at risk for injury. In their data, 27.3% of injuries affected the knee joint, and more than half of injuries required reference to a hospital as a potentially severe injury was suspected. When considering knee injuries alone, they also found that beginners (OR 3.13) were at increased risk, which matches results found by Coury et al. [17]. Alpine skiing was a risk factor for knee injury (OR 1.82) when comparing with other snow sports like snowboarding and telemark.

Ruedl et al. [13] confirm that women are at higher risk for knee and ACL injuries presenting almost double prevalence for this kind of lesions in their data (30.1% in men and 57.4% in women). They report that 93% of knee injuries happened on slopes, and while off-piste skiing had a higher risk injury, it was not at an expense of knee ones. When analyzing by sex, no environmental risk factors for knee injury were found in men, while in women skiing during a snowfall doubled the prevalence on knee injuries compared with injuries of other body parts. Additionally, they found an increased risk when temperature was low (OR 1.6 when skiing at −10°C vs. +2.7°C). Finally, in this study more knee injuries were found in situations of grippy snow in which, as reported by them, this finding is contrary to other literature reporting a higher index on icy snow.

A very interesting study [11] researched the relationship between ACL injury and ski binding failure. In this study 77.9% of ACL-injured patients reported a failure of ski bindings to release. The percentage of failure to release bindings was even higher in female skiers, in skiers injured after a fall backward (vs. a forward fall), and in those who were skiing slow or very slow. There is always a significantly higher percentage of failure to release in patients diagnosed with a complete tear of the anterior cruciate ligament (vs. those with a partial tear), probably because when the ski is not released it acts as a lever at the knee joint for a longer time. Similar results are reported in [12]: bindings only released in 23.8% of knee-injured skiers, with an even worse percentage if only adults (>18 years old) are considered, and 19.3% of binding release among amateur skiers with a knee injury.

5. Discussion

In the elite alpine skiers, there is a high injury rate, especially in knee injuries and ACL. This high prevalence of knee ligament injuries can also be found in amateur skiers, but probably a more aggressive skiing and risk-taking behavior trying to achieve the best results is what explains the higher injury rate in this expert skiers' group. Comparing to studies done in general population, studies in ski racers present better data with more exact diagnostic information and prognosis. ACL and other knee structure injuries present the same incidence in both men and women; this was a surprising finding when taking into account what literature reports about amateur skiers and other high-risk sports for ACL injury: a higher incidence in women. Differences in skiing technique, fitness, behavior, and equipment between elite alpine skiers and amateurs may explain why ACL injury rate is equal in men and women, among ski racers. Whatever the reason is, in our opinion an effort should be made to minimize ACL injury risk in all athlete skiers, as it is a devastating injury that can be the end of the skier's professional career. We found no agreement in the literature about the most dangerous alpine ski discipline for the knee: slalom is characterized for aggressive technique with short turning-radius skis, which may be a risk factor of a knee ligament lesion with a rotational injury mechanism; on the other side, downhill and giant slalom are characterized for higher speeds, which means higher kinetic energy, plus the fact that a longer ski means a greater lever-arm rotational force being transmitted to the knee joint.

Even with the limitations present in studies involving amateur skiers due to their heterogeneity in methodology and limits on precise diagnostic, treatment, and follow-up, we found that the knee joint is the most frequently injured body part, and some studies show there is an increasing trend in ligamentous knee injuries among alpine skiers. Literature found reports that up to half of the injuries are moderate or severe, especially among older skiers, who present a higher injury risk and also a higher risk for serious injury. In our opinion this may be explained by the decrease in physical capabilities associated with aging. Another group at risk for knee injury is the beginner skiers; no explanations for this were found in the literature. In our opinion a poorer technique, bad decision taken related to poorer risk awareness, and probably less knowledge about the correct settings of equipment gear as ski bindings may explain it.

As also found in other sports studies, amateur women have a higher ACL injury risk when skiing. This was found to be supported widely in literature [10–14]. To explain this difference in incidence, we found literature suggesting on a combination of intrinsic factors: anthropometric differences, decreased notch width, augmented articular laxity and muscle (hamstring) flexibility, age, fitness status, and menstruation phases, plus the extrinsic ones such as the type of ski, ski binding setting, slope, and weather. We agree that most probably a combination of anatomic, functional, and extrinsic factors justifies this higher risk. The exact reasons have still to be discovered, but at least we should be able to focus the preventing efforts in the higher injury-risk groups.

We found literature reporting that in 44% of lower extremity injuries (in 44% of MCL injuries and 43% of ACL injuries) skiers were going slow or were stationary, meaning that skiing slowly increments the risk for ACL injury and the risk of bindings fails to release. This last result probably explains the increased ACL injury risk in a fall when skiing slowly, as a lower kinetic energy, should mean a lower injury risk for knee structures.

Skiing in bad weather situations, lower temperature, and/or during a snowfall also were risk factors for knee injury, especially in women. The explanation for this last finding may be the increased risk of cooling which causes a decrease of muscle performance. In [13], there is reference to literature where a 10 times increase in ACL injury risk is reported in bad light conditions and also in case of strong snowfalls (double of risk) probably due to bad visibility plus lower temperatures. In our opinion bad visibility conditions like snowfalls are high-risk situations as it can make the skier to run into bumps able to turn the ski without being able to see and avoid it. This knowledge should be used to warn or even prevent people from skiing in bad weather days.

5.1 ACL biomechanics and injury mechanisms

As multiple articles in the literature report, the ACL is probably the most common injured ligament of the knee in alpine skiers. The second most common injured structure would be the MCL, although not all series agree on this order.

The anterior cruciate ligament is a primary stabilizer of the knee joint, being the main structure to resist tibia anterior translation with respect to the femur. It also restricts tibia internal rotation with knee between 0 and 30° of flexion, prevents hyperextension, and is a secondary stabilizer against the valgus, especially with the knee in extension, when the MCL has a decreasing role.

The medial collateral ligament is the most important knee-stabilizing structure in the medial part of the joint; its main function is to resist the valgus forces and tibia internal rotation and has a secondary role in preventing the anterior translation of the tibia with respect to the femur.

As just seen both ligaments have similar or supplementary functions and are believed to act synergistically. This can explain the prevalence of combined total and partial injuries in skiing and other sports accidents. In other ACL injury high-risk sports, such as soccer, this lesion usually happens when with a foot planted on the ground the player does a sudden deceleration plus external rotation and/or valgus, presenting a twist at the level of the knee joint. Skiing mechanics involve a dual-surface movement [17], and skiers tend to sustain injuries when the ski catches an edge and there is a body torqueing with relation to the knee joint.

A consequence of special mechanics involved in skiing is that several injury mechanisms have been proposed. Shea et al. [12] affirm that injury mechanism in elite and amateur skiers might be different, a point partially supported by other literature when they report different percentages of each injury mechanism in each one of these groups.

In [12], and also in two interesting reviews [7, 21], proposed injury mechanisms are explained; a summary of this is of high interest for a better understanding of knee injuries in skiers:

- Valgus external rotation: after losing balance and shifting the center of gravity forward, the inside edge of the ski touches the ground producing abduction and external rotation of the tibia, while the skier's body advances respect to the knee, creating a valgus force. This mechanism is thought to damage the MCL and the ACL due to the valgus plus the rotation force applied to the knee. The presence of a valgus deformity may also cause a lateral meniscus traumatic tear. This was found to be the most common mechanism of injury in recreational skiers (up to 32.9% of cases) since the generalized use of carving skies [11, 12], and in one publication [12], it was related to high-level amateur skiers. This injury mechanism was found to be related with the failure of ski bindings to release [11].

- Hyperextension internal rotation: occurring in heavy snow, it happens when the ski is slowed while the body keeps advancing forward. Usually, it associates a crossing of ski tips, producing internal rotation and varus force. The forced internal rotation in a probably extended knee is responsible for the ACL injury; as in an extended position, the ACL is the main knee joint restrictor against the internal rotation. This forced movement can also damage lateral structures like the lateral collateral ligament by distraction or the lateral meniscus if it is trapped under the femoral condyle when turning. This is the reported mechanism in 19% of injured skiers.

- Boot-induced anterior drawer: when the skier lands from a jump, the ski tail is the first part to contact the snow causing the body weight to go backward while the leg is driven forward by the boot attached to the ski, applying an anterior force on the tibia. This effect can be increased by a strong quadriceps contraction to avoid a fall. With this mechanism the ACL is putted under great tension to avoid the anterior translation of the tibia with respect to the femur causing the injury. As the ACL is isolated and there is no rotation or varus-valgus deforming forces, the MCL and other knee structures remain unharmed. This mechanism was reported as the one responsible for only 7.8% of ACL injuries in amateur skiers [12], but it seems to be the most frequent mechanism in elite skiers [4]. Ski bindings are not designed to release when a backward-directed force is applied in the absence of rotational forces, so in this mechanism bindings will not release.

- Phantom foot: it happens when the skier losses balance and falls backward on the rear part of skis, placing the hips below the knees with all body weight on the downhill ski, which internally rotates the knee in hyperflexion. Knee hyperflexion puts the ACL under strain, which facilitates its injury due to the forced rotation. The MCL is also injured, as it is the main restrictor structure against internal rotation in the flexed knee. The fact that all body weight is on this ski makes the lateral meniscus vulnerable to injury as it can get trapped under the turning femoral condyle with axial load. This was reported as the most frequent mechanism before the introduction of carving skis [11], and a recent study reports a 22.5% of cases caused by this mechanism, being the second most frequent in skiers between 30 and 40 years old [12]. There is no agreement in literature about the influence of ski binding's failure to release in these cases.

In elite skiers another two mechanisms have been described:

- Dynamic snowplow: with the weight backward and skis in split position, the unweighted ski forces the knee in valgus and internal rotation. It is believed to be the cause of 15% of ACL injury. It has big similarities with the hyperextension mechanism. The ACL, and also the MCL, limits knee valgus and internal rotation, so in this mechanism both structures are under strain and vulnerable to injury.

- Slip and catch: it is very similar to the previous one but is considered more frequent. This happens during a turn, after losing contact with the snow by the outer ski; when it recovers the ski catches the edge causing rapid flexion, internal rotation, and valgus. A very important reported fact is that in 100% of slip-catch ACL injuries in athletes ski bindings do not release or are release after the injury took place [7].

These two mechanisms are believed to be related with the use of more aggressive and smaller turn radius skis like the ones used in slalom races; even some authors suggest that carving skies (shorter, wider in tip and tail, easier to turn) may augment the injury risk as their design may increase kinetic energy in slopes [7], although this last point is controversial [12].

5.2 Associated injuries

When an ACL injury occurs, other knee joint structures may be at risk, as up to 68% of skiers with an ACL injury present a lesion of another knee joint structure.

If, as seen before, a valgus force is present in the injury mechanism, the medial collateral ligament will probably suffer a tear; the rate of associated ACL + MCL injury has been reported between 16 and 57% [21]. The isolated MCL injury is caused by a direct valgus load of the knee. A problem exist in preventing these injuries, as ski bindings are designed to release when falling forward or when rotating force is applied, so no releasing mechanism exists in cases of isolated valgus torque.

In alpine skiing, the most commonly affected menisci is the lateral. This is reported to be found in 23–55% of ACL-injured knees. Some authors [2, 21] tried to explain the lower incidence of menisci lesions in ACL-injured knees when comparing to other ACL injury high-risk sports. The fact that some injury mechanisms are caused by forces that do not contain rotation or valgus may explain that. Another point is that, contrary to soccer or basketball, at the moment of injury in skiing there can be a distraction of the knee joint and by that not loading the meniscus and saving it from tears and less secondary trauma to the joint. Independent of the cause of a lower incidence of menisci, cartilage, and other joint structure injuries, this is a positive point, as all these lesions can be responsible for the onset of early osteoarthritis in young and active patients.

In two literature reviews, we found contradictory affirmations about the trends in tibia plateau fractures, associated or not with ACL injury. In [3], authors report the finding of a rise in tibia plateau fractures, almost in all cases affecting the anterior part of the lateral plateau (Schatzker I, II, and III fractures) caused by valgus axial forces. In an opposite direction point, the results found in [21] report a 92% decrease in tibia plateau fractures from 1970 to 2003. In our literature review, reports about fractures affecting the knee joint are very scarce, and even some articles are done in ski resort clinics without RX; others are done in hospitals with all diagnostic methods available. In our opinion, it is very improbable that a tibia plateau fracture can go undiagnosed as the injured skier would not be able to go to his home hospital, a situation much more probable to happen in cases of minor injuries or even moderate to severe knee sprains.

A conclusion present in the vast majority of literature reviewed is the low prevalence in ankle and lower leg injuries in adult skiers, either amateur or elite athletes. Ankle and tibia diaphysis fractures were once the most feared and frequent injuries; but there are [3] reports of a 92% decrease in ankle fractures and sprains and up to 80% decrease in tibia fractures since the 1970s.

A general agreement is found in the literature and is also of our opinion that the reason for such a decrease in lower leg injuries while knee injury rates have grown or at least maintained is the change in the skier's equipment. Back in the 1960–1970s, ski boots were made of leather, shorter, and soft-shelled. It is evident that a major change has occurred; nowadays, boots are made of plastic, hard-shelled, and much higher than before. Ski is still a high-risk sports, with falls with or without collision being very frequent; and the kinetic energy of the fall is the same than it was 30–40 years ago. With actual equipment these forces bypass the ankle joint and the leg with all the energy absorbed and dissipated at the knee joint's level. In the authors' opinion, the sole fact of the existence of an injury mechanism called "boot-induced anterior drawer" should be enough to prove this point.

Another gear part that has had major improvements in quality is ski bindings. It is very probable that these changes also played a role in the decrease of lower leg fractures and are considered as key safety equipment. Ski bindings are designed to release when there is a fall forward with or without body rotation (reproducing the most frequent injury mechanisms) but are not done to free the skier's foot in case of a backward fall. In our opinion this is a big design deficiency that has to be fixed soon if there is a will to make skiing a safer sports. The problem now is that, as explained previously, several articles report high percentages of ski binding failure to release, especially linked to some injury mechanisms. In our opinion these equipment failures' high rates are to be considered unacceptable, and efforts have to be made to keep improving with the goal of reducing skiing injuries, particularly those affecting the knee joint.

5.3 Treatment

When considering the management and treatment of knee skiing injuries, the first thing that surprised us is that the majority of authors made no reference to it. Publications using small ski resort clinics, some of them without physician and/or diagnostic tools, admit its limitations and explain their procedure for referring patients with a suspected severe injury to hospitals. In other cases, with data obtained from these near hospitals, great treatment and follow-up evolution are lost when referring the patient for definitive treatment to his/her home hospital [14]. A limitation present in both study types is that of skiers with minor or moderate injuries that do not seek medical attention or that do it later in their home hospital.

Only in [1] et al. report the time loss after an ACL injury in elite skiers, but many times this is a population group with big differences in treatment strategies and goals.

Nowadays, the gold standard treatment for an ACL complete tear in a relatively young and active patient is its reconstruction. Debate about the better technique (mono- vs. bifascicular reconstruction, type of graft, graft fixation, etc.) is a topic outside this review's objectives.

It is also generally accepted that the treatment for an isolated MCL injury is a conservative treatment, which is thought to heal without sequels. There is less evidence about the best treatment of ACL and MCL combined injury.

Some surgeons affirm that the best method is to treat each injury in its gold standard way: surgical reconstruction of the ACL and conservative treatment for the MCL. Others argue that in a combined injury an anterior and valgus instability is present and that for this reason the MCL will not heal properly in the presence of an injured ACL. To solve this problem, there are two options, an operative reconstruction of all injured structures and an early surgery for ACL treatment, which would allow for a successful MCL non-operative treatment.

In our opinion, the majority of combined injuries should be treated with surgery but only for ACL reconstruction. We do not agree with the idea that an early ACL

DOI: http://dx.doi.org/10.5772/intechopen.83646

reconstruction surgery is needed; in fact, for us a delayed ACL surgery is a better option, waiting until medial stability is recovered. Only in cases with a grade III MCL tear with great knee instability after at least 2 months of MCL tear conservative treatment, we recommend its surgical treatment, with plasty reconstruction of both structures.

6. Conclusion

Alpine skiing is a high-risk sports with an elevated number of people injured every year. Ligamentous knee injuries are among the most common, and it does not seems to be any tendency to decrease its high rate despite changes in attitudes and equipment that have lowered the number of other serious injuries. As seen, the percentage of knee injuries that can be considered severe is high, with ACL tears as the most common knee injury. Having such high rates of serious injuries in alpine skier's knee implies big challenges in prevention, to identify skiers at risk and to improve equipment parts that are proven to be failing. More research needs to be done to define all risk factors so that prevention efforts can be well directed. Also, more research is needed to identify the best treatment option for ACL and other knee ligamentous injuries, and consensus in treatment and rehabilitation protocols are needed for both elite athletes and amateur-injured alpine skiers.

Conflict of interest

Authors declare no conflict of interest.

Author details

Guillem Navarro Escarp[1], Oscar Ares Rodriguez[1,2,3*], Ignacio Moya Molinas[1], Pilar Camacho Carrasco[1,3], Alonso Zumbado Dijeres[1,3], Roberto Seijas Vazquez[4,5], Andrea Sallent[6], Manuel Llusa Pérez[1,3] and Andreu Combalia Aleu[1,3]

1 Hospital Clínic de Barcelona, Barcelona, Spain

2 Centro Médico Teknon, Barcelona, Spain

3 Universitat de Barcelona, Barcelona, Spain

4 Hospital Quiron Barcelona, Barcelona, Spain

5 Universitat Internacional de Catalunya, Barcelona, Spain

6 Hospital Vall d'hebron, Barcelona, Spain

*Address all correspondence to: arestraumatologia@gmail.com

References

[1] Stenroos AJ, Handolin LE. Alpine skiing injuries in Finland—A two-year retrospective study based on a questionnaire among ski racers. BMC Sports Science, Medicine and Rehabilitation. 2014;**6**(1):2-6

[2] Patrick E, Cooper JG, Daniels J. Changes in skiing and snowboarding injury epidemiology and attitudes to safety in big sky, Montana, USA: A comparison of 2 cross-sectional studies in 1996 and 2013. Orthopaedic Journal of Sports Medicine. 2015;**3**(6):1-6

[3] Hunter RE. Current concepts skiing injuries. Sports Medicine. 2000;**27**(3):381-389

[4] Flørenes TW, Bere T, Nordsletten L, Heir S, Bahr R. Injuries among male and female world cup alpine skiers. British Journal of Sports Medicine. 2009;**43**(13):973-978

[5] Schmitt K-U, Hörterer N, Vogt M, Frey WO, Lorenzetti S. Investigating physical fitness and race performance as determinants for the ACL injury risk in alpine ski racing. BMC Sports Science, Medicine and Rehabilitation. 2016;**8**(1):23

[6] Bere T, Flørenes TW, Nordsletten L, Bahr R. Sex differences in the risk of injury in world cup alpine skiers: A 6-year cohort study. British Journal of Sports Medicine. 2014;**48**(1):36-40

[7] Jordan M, Aagaard P, Herzog W. Anterior cruciate ligament injury/reinjury in alpine ski racing: A narrative review. Open Access Journal of Sports Medicine. 2017;**8**:71-83

[8] Ruedl G, Philippe M, Sommersacher R, Duennwald T, Kopp M, Burtscher M. Current incidence of accidents on Austrian Ski slopes. Sportverletzung-Sportschaden. 2014;**28**(4):183-187

[9] Girardi P, Braggion M, Sacco G, de Giorgi F, Corra S. Factors affecting injury severity among recreational skiers and snowboarders: An epidemiology study. Knee Surgery, Sport Traumatol Arthrosc. 2010;**18**(12):1804-1809

[10] Khalilifar AH, Kazemi MH, Hamedanchi A, Hosseini MJ. Skiing injuries at the Dizin ski resort. Trauma Monthly. 2012;**17**(1):259-261

[11] Ruedl G, Helle K, Tecklenburg K, Schranz A, Fink C, Burtscher M. Factors associated with self-reported failure of binding release among ACL injured male and female recreational skiers: A catalyst to change ISO binding standards? British Journal of Sports Medicine. 2016;**50**(1):37-40

[12] Shea KG, Archibald-Seiffer N, Murdock E, Grimm NL, Jacobs JC, Willick S, et al. Knee injuries in downhill skiers: A 6-year survey study. Orthopaedic Journal of Sports Medicine. 2014;**2**(1):1-6

[13] Ruedl G, Fink C, Schranz A, Sommersacher R, Nachbauer W, Burtscher M. Impact of environmental factors on knee injuries in male and female recreational skiers. Scandinavian Journal of Medicine & Science in Sports. 2012;**22**(2):185-189

[14] Castellani C, Singer G, Kaiser M, Petnehazy T, et al. An epidemiologic analysis of winter sport accidents on ski slopes comparing two seasons. The Journal of Sports Medicine and Physical Fitness. 2018

[15] Davidson TM, Laliotis AT. Alpine skiing injuries. A nine-year study. The Western Journal of Medicine. 1996;**164**(4):310-314

[16] Warme WJ, John A, King P, Lambert KL, Cunningham RR, Hole J. Injury statistics, 1982-1993 Jackson Hole Ski

Resort. American Journal of Sports Medicine. 1993;**23**(5):597-600

[17] Coury T, Napoli AM, Wilson M, Daniels J, Murray T, Milzman D. Injury patterns in recreational alpine skiing and snowboarding at a mountainside clinic. Wilderness & Environmental Medicine. 2013;**24**(4):417-421

[18] Wasden CC, McIntosh SE, Keith DS, McCowan C. An analysis of skiing and snowboarding injuries on Utah slopes. Journal of Trauma, Injury, Infection, and Critical Care. 2009;**67**(5):1022-1026

[19] Ekeland A, Rødven A, Heir S. Injuries among children and adults in alpine skiing and snowboarding. Journal of Science and Medicine in Sport. 2018:11-14

[20] Sulheim S, Holme I, Rødven A, Ekeland A, Bahr R. Risk factors for injuries in alpine skiing, telemark skiing and snowboarding—Case-control study. British Journal of Sports Medicine. 2011;**45**(16):1303-1309

[21] Pressman A, Johnson DH. A review of ski injuries resulting in combined injury to the anterior cruciate ligament and medial collateral ligaments. Arthroscopy: The Journal of Arthroscopic & Related Surgery. 2003;**19**(2):194-202

Chapter 3

Decision-Making for ALL Reconstruction and Surgical Techniques

Tahsin Gurpinar

Abstract

The anterolateral ligament (ALL), which was first described in 1879, was reintroduced in 2013 by Claes et al. It originates near the lateral epicondyle of the distal femur, runs along the lateral outer aspect of the knee, and inserts on the proximal tibia between Gerdy's tubercle and fibular head. The ALL tightens when the knee is internally rotated (twisted inwards), and in doing so, it is proposed to be a stabilizer to internal tibial rotation. Biomechanical studies showed that the ALL restrains internal rotation of the tibia and thus affects the pivot-shift phenomenon in the anterior cruciate ligament (ACL)-injured knee. Therefore, it is proposed that the deficient ALL can be a reason for persistent rotatory instability after ACL reconstruction. Furthermore, ALL reconstruction techniques have evolved and indications extended. Commonly accepted indications for concomitant ACL and ALL reconstruction are ACL revisions, high-grade pivot-shift test, chronic ACL rupture, and young patients and patients doing pivoting activities. Most surgeons perform an anatomic reconstruction technique with gracilis autograft. However, only few studies published reporting the outcomes of ALL reconstruction and more studies with longer follow-up times are, therefore, needed to provide the compelling clinical evidence for the efficacy of concomitant ACL and ALL procedures.

Keywords: anterolateral ligament, ALL reconstruction,
indications for ALL reconstruction, anterior cruciate ligament, pivot shift

1. Introduction

The anterolateral ligament (ALL) is a newly re-introduced ligament on the lateral aspect of the knee, which originates at the lateral epicondyle of the femur, and inserts at the anterolateral aspect of the proximal tibia. It was first described by Paul Segond as "a pearly, resistant, fibrous band" at the anterolateral aspect of the human knee; however, it was not given much importance until Claes et al. identified the ALL in an anatomic study as a distinct structure of the lateral compartment of the knee [1]. Subsequently, many studies have been published regarding the anatomy, biomechanics, and radiology of ALL.

The clinical relevance of ALL mostly comes from its high association with anterior cruciate ligament (ACL) injuries. Studies showed a high incidence of radiological ALL damage (78.7%) in ACL-injured knees [2]. Biomechanically, it is claimed to be a stabilizer in internal rotation of the tibia particularly at high knee flexion

IntechOpen

angles; however, the biomechanical role of ALL is still the subject of debate [3, 4]. This chapter reviews the main features related to ALL and focuses on the current indications and techniques of ALL reconstruction.

2. Anatomy

The anatomy of the ALL has been investigated by several authors in order to accurately identify the features of the structure. There has been some debate regarding the exact attachments of the ligament; however, it is generally accepted that the ALL is a distinctive triangular, anterolateral structure under the iliotibial band (ITB). Investigations of the anatomy of the ALL in several cadavers have revealed variability of the structure particularly for the femoral attachment. The femoral origin is located at the lateral femoral epicondyle (LFE) at either the identical position of the origin of the fibular collateral ligament (FCL) or just posterior and proximal to it with the average width at this point 11.85 mm [5]. The ALL then runs distally by overlapping the proximal portion of the lateral collateral ligament, and some fibers of the ALL are attached to the lateral meniscus and the anterolateral capsule at the level of knee joint. The majority of the fibers continue to run distally and attach midway between the tip of the fibular head and GT (**Figure 1**). The tibial attachment is 12.2 ± 3.0 mm width and is centered 21.6 mm posterior to Gerdy's tubercle, and 4–10 mm far from the joint line [1, 6–8]. The mean length of the structure has been measured between 34 and 59 mm from its femoral origin to tibial attachment [7, 8]. The thickness of ALL also varies and has been measured as 2.09 mm in males and 1.09 mm in females [9].

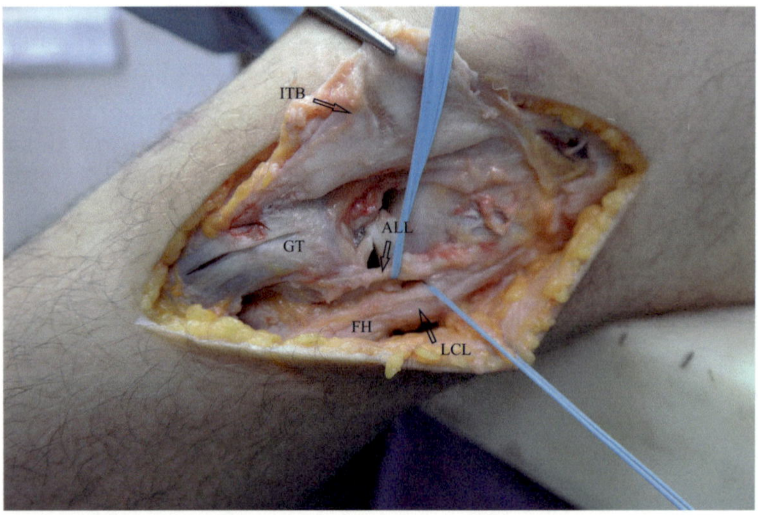

Figure 1.
Anterolateral ligament anatomy (ITB: iliotibial band, ALL: anterolateral ligament, FH: fibular head, GT: Gerdy's tubercle, and LCL: lateral collateral ligament).

3. Biomechanics

Zens et al. [10] found that the isolated ALL had an ultimate tensile strength of 50 ± 15 N, at a strain of 36 ± 4%. With a mean cross-sectional area of only 1.54 mm^2, the ultimate tensile stress was 33 ± 4 MPa and the overall stiffness was 4.2 N/mm extension. However, Kennedy et al. [11] reported that the ALL had a tensile strength of 175 N (139–211 N 95% CI) and stiffness 20 N/mm [12–21] with a more substantial structure than that shown by Zens et al. [10]. The mean ultimate load to failure and the mean stiffness of ALL have been measured between 50 and 205 N and between 20 and 42 N/mm, respectively, in different studies [11, 22, 23].

In most of the studies, the ALL is described as a secondary stabilizer to internal rotation and to some extent anterior translation [3, 24, 25]. The biomechanical studies demonstrated that in the presence of ACL deficiency, sectioning the ALL in cadaveric specimens significantly effects the anteroposterior (AP) stability as well as results in a significant increase in internal rotation [12, 24]. The contribution of the ALL during internal rotation increases significantly with increasing flexion, whereas that of the ACL decreased significantly. Therefore, it is speculated that the ALL deficiency can be a reason for persistent rotational instability after ACL reconstruction [13].

The isometry of the ALL was measured by Dodds et al. [7], by threading a suture along the ligament fibers, attaching it to the moving tibia and then measuring the changes of the separation distance between the attachments using a transducer. It was shown that the ALL was not isometric, but was close to being isometric from 0 to 60° knee flexion. Internal tibial rotation increased the length between the attachments, and external rotation reduced it. When the knee was in extension, tibial rotations in response to 5 Nm torque were not large enough to cause significant change in the length of the ALL. However, internal tibial rotation increased the mean length between the ALL attachments from 3.6 mm (SD 0.7; 1.5–5.7) at 30° ($p = 0.003$) to 9.9 mm (SD 1.4; 5.7–14.2) at 90° of flexion of the knee. Imbert et al. [14] investigated isometric characteristics of the ALL in a cadaveric navigation study and found that ALL is not isometric at any of the femoral insertion locations but had different length change patterns during knee flexion and internal tibial rotation at 90°. However, they found that the proximal and posterior to epicondyle femoral position is favorable to being isometry.

4. Injury

Injury to the ALL is most commonly associated with a concomitant tear of the ACL. In a retrospective MRI study, Claes et al. [2] analyzed 206 ACL injured knees and found 78.8% radiological ALL abnormalities. Most of the ALL abnormalities were found to be situated in the distal part of the ligament (77.8%), whereas 20.4% of the injuries were proximal and only 1.8% knees were diagnosed with a bony ALL avulsion. Ferretti et al. [15] exposed the lateral knee compartments of 60 patients undergoing ACLR and found several lesion types of the ALL injuries including macroscopic hemorrhage extending to the anterolateral capsule (32%) or to the posterolateral capsule (27%), complete transverse tear of the ALL near its tibial insertion (22%), and a bony tibial avulsion (Segond fracture) (10%). In a retrospective MRI study, Gurpinar et al. found 65.2% ALL injury in patients underwent ACL surgery who were diagnosed with isolated ACL injury previously [13]. In a similar study, van Dyck et al. [16] found ALL abnormalities in 46% of 90 knee MRIs of patients with an acute ACL rupture. Furthermore, they found that these patients were more likely to have a lateral meniscal tear, collateral ligament injury, or osseous injury compared with patients with an intact ALL.

After re-discovery of ALL, Segond fractures, which were previously considered as a diagnostic clue for ACL injury, are classified as ALL equivalent injuries [17]. Porrino et al. [18] evaluated 20 knee MRIs with a Segond fracture and found that the ALL was attached to the fracture fragment in all but one case limited by anatomic distortion. Claes et al. [17] also suggested that the Segond fracture is actually a bony avulsion of the ALL. However, Shaikh et al. [19] claimed that ITB and lateral capsule attached to the Segond fracture in 94% of the patients and Segond fracture is not merely an ALL avulsion but the avulsion of the anterolateral complex.

On the other hand, anterolateral injuries and instability can also occur in the ACL intact states. Gottsegen et al. [20] and DeLee et al. [21] reported the Segond fracture combined to popliteal tendon avulsion and iliotibial band avulsion. Wharton et al. [26] published a case report in which the Segond fracture was combined to posterolateral ligament injury without ACL rupture. Furthermore, Ferreira reported an absolute isolated Segond fracture.

5. Diagnosis

Diagnosing ALL lesions can be difficult since no specific clinical tests have been validated for the diagnosis of ALL injuries. To achieve an impeccable diagnosis, meticulous clinical examination and appropriate evaluation of the radiographic and MRI imaging are necessary. Since ALL is highly associated with ACL injury, patients subjected to trauma mechanisms similar to an isolated ACL injury such as contact and noncontact injuries involving early flexion, dynamic valgus, and internal rotation should also be suspected for ALL injury. Anterior drawer and Lachman tests can be positive due to the concomitant ACL injury. However, since ALL is primarily responsible for rotational stability, pivot-shift test is considered to be the most reliable test to evaluate ALL integrity. Monaco et al. [27] demonstrated that a grade III pivot shift is only seen in the absence of both the ACL and ALL in vitro. However, the potential confusing factors of a high-grade pivot shift, such as a lateral meniscus or root tear, ITB injury, or general hyperlaxity should be assessed [28, 29].

Segond fracture is also considered to be ALL avulsion, and therefore, it can be assumed that symptoms related to a Segond fracture may be present in ALL injury including provoked pain on palpation of the lateral tibia or increased laxity in varus stress. On examination, the lateral compartment of the knee should be carefully evaluated, and the integrity of the cruciate and collateral ligaments should be examined too. However, in the acute phase, diagnosis can be challenging and evaluation should be repeated in subacute and chronic phases after swelling and pain has decreased.

6. Surgical indications

The optimal ACL reconstruction is still a debate in orthopedic research, and persistent rotatory instability has been reported up to 25% of cases after an isolated ACL reconstruction procedure [30]. Some studies found that an isolated ACL reconstruction can control the translational instability, but is insufficient to restore the normal rotational stability. In addition, the persistent rotatory instability does not only cause difficulties with pivoting sports, but also can cause secondary meniscal and cartilaginous problems [31]. Furthermore, younger and higher-level athletes with rotational instability can be vulnerable to re-ruptures. Therefore, combining a lateral extra-articular procedure with an intra-articular reconstruction for the treatment of ACL injury emerged, with the aim of decreasing rotational instability. However, long-term results of ALL reconstruction are not known and have not been suggested as a standard procedure with ACL reconstruction. Despite this, additional ALL reconstruction has been recommended in patients with grade III pivot shift or Segond fracture and athletes practicing of sports with pivot movements [32–34]. In addition ACL revision, subjective rotational looseness, and Telos value >10 mm are also considered as indicative of ALL reconstruction associated with ACL reconstruction [35]. Some surgeons also suggested ALL reconstruction in cases of chronic ACL reconstruction, high level of sports activity, and radiographic lateral femoral notch sign [36].

Recently the ALL Expert Group [37] proposed a decision tree for the management of ACL ruptures and recommended ALL reconstruction for patients who present at least: (1) decisive criteria for increased risk of secondary ACL rupture or postoperative residual positive pivot shift or (2) secondary criteria for increased risk of secondary ACL rupture or postoperative residual positive pivot shift including history, clinical or imaging signs, or patient profile. However, literature still lacks good-quality randomized studies and more studies are needed to prove these findings.

7. Reconstruction

7.1 Graft type and preparation

Wytrykowski et al. [38] performed a cadaveric study to compare the biomechanical properties of the ALL, gracilis, and IT band. The gracilis was found to have six times the stiffness of the ALL (131.7 vs. 21 N/mm) and had the highest maximum load to failure (200.7 vs. 141 N). The mechanical properties of the IT band (stiffness, 39.9 N/mm; maximum load to failure, 161.1 N) most closely resembled those of the ALL. However, many authors have published techniques using a gracilis graft for ALL reconstruction and a tripled semitendinosus auto- or allograft or quadrupled semitendinosus autograft with all-inside technique for the reconstruction of ACL [39–41]. The use of polyester tape [42] or a single-bundle semitendinosus auto- or allograft has also been described in the literature [43]. In our clinic, we use gracilis graft for ALL reconstruction, and for the ACL, we use quadriceps autograft, tripled semitendinosus, or allograft.

7.2 Femoral and tibial origins and fixation

On the tibia, the anatomical landmarks are the center of the fibula head, the center of Gerdy's tubercle, and joint line (**Figure 2a**). We use the midpoint between Gerdy's tubercle and the fibula at 5–10 mm below the lateral joint line for the site of tibial fixation. We make a stab incision 5–10 mm below the joint line, halfway between the center of Gerdy's tubercle and the fibula head (**Figure 2b**). Helito et al. [44] have described the radiographic landmarks to determine this location. They choose a point around 7 mm below the tibial plateau on the AP view and around 50% of the plateau length on the lateral view [39]. Similar tibial attachment points have been used by many authors; however, some surgeons used two attachment points, and therefore, they used one point just anterior to the fibular head and second point posterior to the Gerdy's tubercle [45].

Since the origin of the femoral insertion of the ALL varies, the location of femoral fixation during ALLR is a debate. Many authors [40, 46, 47] described a fixation at a point posterior and superior to the lateral femoral epicondyle; however, some [41, 42] described a fixation slightly anterior to the lateral epicondyle. As a radiological reference point, Helito et al. used Blumensaat's line and identified the femoral attachment at approximately halfway along Blumensaat's line from the anterior edge of the femoral condyle [44]. Kennedy et al. used the intersection of two lines: one was the parallel extension of the posterior femoral cortex and the second line was drawn perpendicularly to the first line and intersecting the most

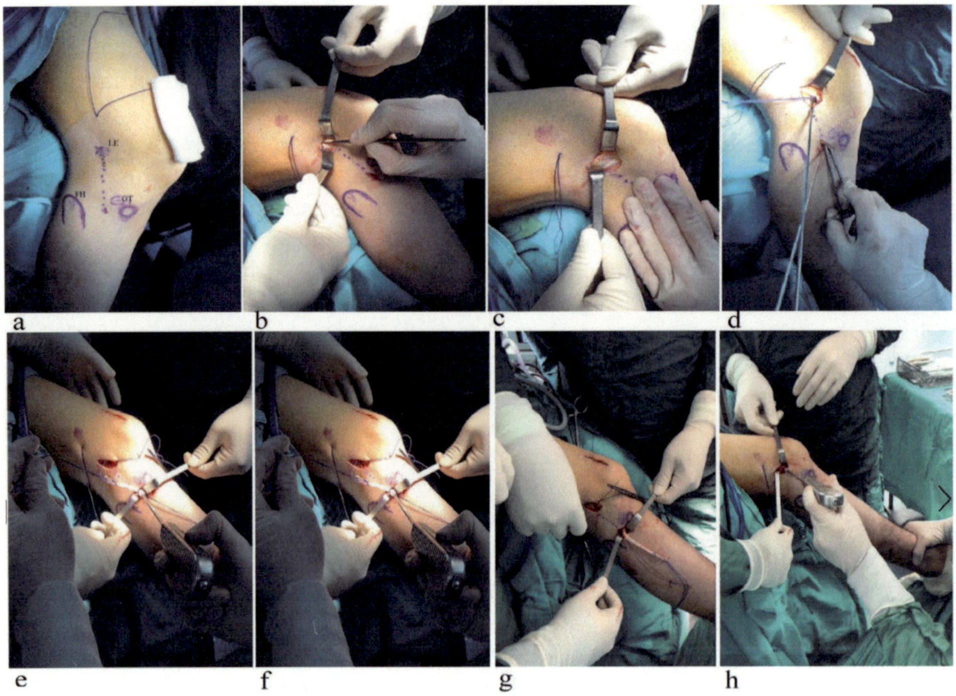

Figure 2.
Step-by-step anterolateral ligament reconstruction.

posterior aspect of Blumensaat's line [11]. In our clinic, we make a 5–10 mm incision just proximal to the epicondyle, and after dividing the ITB, we insert the drill pin slightly proximal and posterior to the lateral epicondyle (**Figure 1c** and **d**).

After inserting femoral and tibial pin guides, the passing suture is placed under the ITB around the femoral wire and tibial wires. The knee is then moved through the full range of motion (**Figure 1d**). The isometry assessment is made to be sure that the graft will not tighten in flexion and will be tight in extension. If the suture tightens in flexion, the femoral socket may be too distal or anterior.

After the isometry test, the graft is passed under the ITB and fixed with interference screws or anchors on both sides, while the knee is 30° flexed and at neutral rotation (**Figure 2**). However, fixation in full extension at 45–60° of flexion or fixation at 60–90° of flexion have also been described in the literature [39, 40, 47]. Different surgical techniques and indications are summarized in **Table 1**.

8. Postoperative rehabilitation

The plaster cast immobilization or bracing were popular in the historical literature when ACL and lateral extra-articular procedures were performed together [49]. However, use of brace is much less common in current practice. Many authors recommend that rehabilitation after an additional ALL reconstruction should be carried out in a similar way compared to isolated ACL rehabilitation. An early aggressive rehabilitation program can be applied. Emphasis should be placed on achieving symmetrical full knee extension, decreasing knee joint effusion, and quadriceps activation early in the rehabilitation process. Passive flexion and patellar mobilization, avoiding eccentric quadriceps contraction, should also be performed. Weight bearing as tolerated is recommended immediately following surgery to promote knee extension and hinder quadriceps inhibition.

DOI: http://dx.doi.org/10.5772/intechopen.86398

Author/ year	Reported indications	Graft types	Femoral fixation point	Tibial fixation point	Fixation types	Fixation angle
Helito et al. [39]	High-grade pivot-shift examination, ACL revision without apparent cause for failure	Gracilis	3–4 mm below the halfway point on the Blumensaat's line in the AP direction	5–10 mm below the lateral tibial plateau	Inference screw 1 size greater than tunnel diameter	60–90° of flexion
Smith et al. [41]	Marked laxity on examination under anesthesia	Gracilis	Anterior to lateral femoral epicondyle	Midway between fibular head and the Gerdy's tubercle, 11 mm distal to joint line	5.5-mm suture anchors	30° of flexion
Sonnery-Cottet et al. [47]	Segond fractures, chronic ACL tears, grade III pivot shift, high-level or pivot sports participation, lateral femoral notch sign	Gracilis	Proximal and posterior to lateral epicondyle	Site of Segond fracture, at tibial footprint of ALL	4.75 or 5.5 mm interference screw	Not reported
Ferreira et al. [40]	Asymmetry of lateral plateau with internal rotation, grade II/III pivot shift, ALL tear on MRI, Segond fractures	Gracilis	8 mm posterosuperiorly from lateral epicondyle	9–13 mm distal to lateral joint line	Interference screw 2 mm larger than tunnel	45–60° flexion
Chahla et al. [43]	Grade III pivot shift, multiple ACL reconstructions with residual laxity, clinically significant instability after ACL reconstruction	Semitendinosus	4.7 mm proximal and posterior to FCL insertion site	Midway between the Gerdy's tubercle and anterior margin fibular head (9.5 mm distal to joint line)	7 × 28-mm interference screw	30° flexion
Wagih and Elguindy [42]	Grade III pivot-shift examination	Polyester tape	Anterior and distal to lateral femoral condyle	Midpoint between the Gerdy's tubercle and the fibular head	Cortical suspension button	30° flexion
Saithna et al. [45]	Young age (<20 years old). Participation in pivoting sports or a high-demand athlete, high-grade pivot shift on examination, lateral femoral notch sign on preoperative imaging, Segond fracture. Revision ACL reconstruction. Chronic (>12 months) ACL injury	Gracilis	Just proximal and posterior to the lateral epicondyle	One point just anterior to the fibular head and second posterior to Gerdy's tubercle	Tibial tunnel no fixation femoral side ACL graft ethibond	Full extension

Author/ year	Reported indications	Graft types	Femoral fixation point	Tibial fixation point	Fixation types	Fixation angle
Delaloye et al. [48]	ACL repair	Gracilis	Posterior and proximal to the lateral epicondyle	One point just anterior to the fibular head and second posterior to Gerdy's tubercle	SwiveLock anchor	Full extension

Table 1.
Indications, femoral and tibial fixation points, and fixation materials and angles reported in the literature.

9. Clinical outcomes

To date, only few studies reported the clinical outcomes of ALL reconstruction since the rediscovery of this ligament [32, 33, 36, 50]. In a retrospective case series, Sonnery-Cottet et al. [36] evaluated 92 patients at a minimum 2-year follow-up after concomitant ACL and ALL reconstruction. Compared with the preoperative assessment, the follow-up showed significant improvements in Lysholm score, subjective IKDC score, and objective IKDC score. Pivot-shift results were also significantly improved; however, this study did not have a control group.

In a prospective comparative study of 502 patients, Sonnery et al. found lower graft rupture rate with combined ALL-ACL reconstruction technique in a high-risk population, compared to the isolated ACL reconstructions that used a bone-patellar tendon-bone graft or a quadrupled hamstring tendon graft [33]. Another randomized study showed an improvement in knee laxity measured using a KT-1000 arthrometer in patients with combined ACL and ALL reconstructions compared to patients with isolated ACL reconstructions; however, the other measured parameters did not differ significantly [32]. Recently, Helito et al. [50] evaluated the results of combined ACL-ALL reconstruction with isolated ACL reconstruction in 101 chronic ACL injuries. Regarding functional outcome scores, they found better results on both the IKDC and the Lysholm evaluations in combined ACL-ALL reconstruction group. In addition, patients in the ACL-ALL reconstruction group had better KT-1000 evaluation and a lower pivot-shift rate at physical examination. Although the results of the recent studies are promising, indications for ALL reconstruction are not identical in these studies and additional studies are needed to confirm these results.

10. Conclusions

In conclusion, it is commonly accepted that the ALL is a distinctive structure that originates from proximal and posterior to the femoral epicondyle, attaches slightly posterior to the Gerdy's tubercle, and functions as a secondary stabilizer to internal rotation. In addition, it has been reported that it has a crucial role in preventing pivot-shift phenomenon. However, there is a lack of evidence supporting that it can be a reason for persistent pivot shift after ACL reconstructions [13]. Although the results of the recent studies reporting the outcomes of ALL reconstruction are promising, the total volume of literature on this topic is limited and composed of low-quality evidence. More studies with longer follow-up times are, therefore, needed to provide the convincing clinical evidence for the favor of concomitant ACL and ALL procedures. In addition, despite the lack of clear evidence for an increase in lateral compartment osteoarthritis after concomitant procedures, compression in the lateral compartment seems to be a concern and was regarded as a reason to abandon concomitant lateral procedures historically [51–53].

Acknowledgements

There is no support funding for the publication.

Conflict of interest

The author declares that no conflict of interest exists.

Author details

Tahsin Gurpinar
University of Health Sciences, Istanbul Research and Education Hospital, Istanbul, Turkey

*Address all correspondence to: tahsingurpinar@msn.com

References

[1] Claes S, Vereecke E, Maes M, Victor J, Verdonk P, Bellemans J. Anatomy of the anterolateral ligament of the knee. Journal of Anatomy. 2013;**223**(4):321-328

[2] Claes S, Bartholomeeusen S, Bellemans J. High prevalence of anterolateral ligament abnormalities in magnetic resonance images of anterior cruciate ligament-injured knees. Acta Orthopaedica Belgica. 2014;**80**(1):45-49

[3] Parsons EM, Gee AO, Spiekerman C, Cavanagh PR. The biomechanical function of the anterolateral ligament of the knee. The American Journal of Sports Medicine. 2015;**43**(3):669-674

[4] Guenther D, Rahnemai-Azar AA, Fu FH, Debski RE. The biomechanical function of the anterolateral ligament of the knee: Letter to the editor. The American Journal of Sports Medicine. 2015;**43**(8):NP21-NP22

[5] Daggett M, Ockuly AC, Cullen M, Busch K, Lutz C, Imbert P, et al. Femoral origin of the anterolateral ligament: An anatomic analysis. Arthroscopy. 2016;**32**(5):835-841

[6] Caterine S, Litchfield R, Johnson M, Chronik B, Getgood A. A cadaveric study of the anterolateral ligament: Re-introducing the lateral capsular ligament. Knee Surgery, Sports Traumatology, Arthroscopy. 2015;**23**(11):3186-3195

[7] Dodds AL, Halewood C, Gupte CM, Williams A, Amis AA. The anterolateral ligament: Anatomy, length changes and association with the Segond fracture. The Bone & Joint Journal. 2014;**96-B**(3):325-331

[8] Vincent JP, Magnussen RA, Gezmez F, Uguen A, Jacobi M, Weppe F, et al. The anterolateral ligament of the human knee: An anatomic and histologic study. Knee Surgery, Sports Traumatology, Arthroscopy. 2012;**20**(1):147-152

[9] Daggett M, Busch K, Sonnery-Cottet B. Surgical dissection of the anterolateral ligament. Arthroscopy Techniques. 2016;**5**(1):e185-e188

[10] Zens M, Feucht MJ, Ruhhammer J, Bernstein A, Mayr HO, Südkamp NP, et al. Mechanical tensile properties of the anterolateral ligament. Journal of Experimental Orthopaedics. 2015;**2**(1):7

[11] Kennedy MI, Claes S, Fuso FA, Williams BT, Goldsmith MT, Turnbull TL, et al. The anterolateral ligament: An anatomic, radiographic, and biomechanical analysis. The American Journal of Sports Medicine. 2015;**43**(7):1606-1615

[12] Ruiz N, Filippi GJ, Gagnière B, Bowen M, Robert HE. The comparative role of the anterior cruciate ligament and anterolateral structures in controlling passive internal rotation of the knee: A biomechanical study. Arthroscopy. 2016;**32**(6):1053-1062

[13] Gürpınar T, Polat B, Polat AE, Mutlu İ, Tüzüner T. Is anterolateral ligament rupture a reason for persistent rotational instability after anterior cruciate ligament reconstruction? The Knee. 2018;**25**(6):1033-1039

[14] Imbert P, Lutz C, Daggett M, Niglis L, Freychet B, Dalmay F, et al. Isometric characteristics of the anterolateral ligament of the knee: A cadaveric navigation study. Arthroscopy. 2016;**32**(10):2017-2024

[15] Ferretti A, Monaco E, Fabbri M, Maestri B, De Carli A. Prevalence and classification of injuries of anterolateral complex in acute anterior cruciate ligament tears. Arthroscopy. 2017;**33**(1):147-154

[16] Van Dyck P, Clockaerts S, Vanhoenacker FM, Lambrecht V, Wouters K, De Smet E, et al. Anterolateral ligament abnormalities in patients with acute anterior cruciate ligament rupture are associated with lateral meniscal and osseous injuries. European Radiology. 2016;**26**(10):3383-3391

[17] Claes S, Luyckx T, Vereecke E, Bellemans J. The Segond fracture: A bony injury of the anterolateral ligament of the knee. Arthroscopy. 2014;**30**(11):1475-1482

[18] Porrino J, Maloney E, Richardson M, Mulcahy H, Ha A, Chew FS. The anterolateral ligament of the knee: MRI appearance, association with the Segond fracture, and historical perspective. AJR. American Journal of Roentgenology. 2015;**204**(2):367-373

[19] Shaikh H, Herbst E, Rahnemai-Azar AA, Bottene Villa Albers M, Naendrup JH, Musahl V, et al. The Segond fracture is an avulsion of the anterolateral complex. The American Journal of Sports Medicine. 2017;**45**(10):2247-2252

[20] Gottsegen CJ, Eyer BA, White EA, Learch TJ, Forrester D. Avulsion fractures of the knee: Imaging findings and clinical significance. Radiographics. 2008;**28**(6):1755-1770

[21] DeLee JC, Riley MB, Rockwood CA. Acute posterolateral rotatory instability of the knee. The American Journal of Sports Medicine. 1983;**11**(4):199-207

[22] Helito CP, Bonadio MB, Rozas JS, Wey JM, Pereira CA, Cardoso TP, et al. Biomechanical study of strength and stiffness of the knee anterolateral ligament. BMC Musculoskeletal Disorders. 2016;**17**:193

[23] Zens M, Niemeyer P, Ruhhammer J, Bernstein A, Woias P, Mayr HO, et al. Length changes of the anterolateral ligament during passive knee motion: A human cadaveric study. The American Journal of Sports Medicine. 2015;**43**(10):2545-2552

[24] Rasmussen MT, Nitri M, Williams BT, Moulton SG, Cruz RS, Dornan GJ, et al. An in vitro robotic assessment of the anterolateral ligament, part 1: Secondary role of the anterolateral ligament in the setting of an anterior cruciate ligament injury. The American Journal of Sports Medicine. 2016;**44**(3):585-592

[25] Schon JM, Moatshe G, Brady AW, Serra Cruz R, Chahla J, Dornan GJ, et al. Anatomic anterolateral ligament reconstruction of the knee leads to overconstraint at any fixation angle. The American Journal of Sports Medicine. 2016;**44**(10):2546-2556

[26] Wharton R, Henckel J, Bhattee G, Ball S, Church S. Segond fracture in an adult is not pathognomonic for ACL injury. Knee Surgery, Sports Traumatology, Arthroscopy. 2015;**23**(7):1925-1928

[27] Monaco E, Ferretti A, Labianca L, Maestri B, Speranza A, Kelly MJ, et al. Navigated knee kinematics after cutting of the ACL and its secondary restraint. Knee Surgery, Sports Traumatology, Arthroscopy. 2012;**20**(5):870-877

[28] Song GY, Zhang H, Liu X, Zhang J, Xue Z, Qian Y, et al. Complete posterolateral meniscal root tear is associated with high-grade pivot-shift phenomenon in noncontact anterior cruciate ligament injuries. Knee Surgery, Sports Traumatology, Arthroscopy. 2017;**25**(4):1030-1037

[29] Tanaka M, Vyas D, Moloney G, Bedi A, Pearle AD, Musahl V. What does it take to have a high-grade pivot shift? Knee Surgery, Sports Traumatology, Arthroscopy. 2012;**20**(4):737-742

[30] Chouliaras V, Ristanis S, Moraiti C, Tzimas V, Stergiou N, Georgoulis AD.

Anterior cruciate ligament reconstruction with a quadrupled hamstrings tendon autograft does not restore tibial rotation to normative levels during landing from a jump and subsequent pivoting. The Journal of Sports Medicine and Physical Fitness. 2009;**49**(1):64-70

[31] Stergiou N, Ristanis S, Moraiti C, Georgoulis AD. Tibial rotation in anterior cruciate ligament (ACL)-deficient and ACL-reconstructed knees: A theoretical proposition for the development of osteoarthritis. Sports Medicine. 2007;**37**(7):601-613

[32] Ibrahim SA, Shohdy EM, Marwan Y, Ramadan SA, Almisfer AK, Mohammad MW, et al. Anatomic reconstruction of the anterior cruciate ligament of the knee with or without reconstruction of the anterolateral ligament: A randomized clinical trial. The American Journal of Sports Medicine. 2017;**45**(7):1558-1566

[33] Sonnery-Cottet B, Saithna A, Cavalier M, Kajetanek C, Temponi EF, Daggett M, et al. Anterolateral ligament reconstruction is associated with significantly reduced ACL graft rupture rates at a minimum follow-up of 2 years: A prospective comparative study of 502 patients from the SANTI study group. The American Journal of Sports Medicine. 2017;**45**(7):1547-1557

[34] Zhang H, Qiu M, Zhou A, Zhang J, Jiang D. Anatomic anterolateral ligament reconstruction improves postoperative clinical outcomes combined with anatomic anterior cruciate ligament reconstruction. Journal of Sports Science and Medicine. 2016;**15**(4):688-696

[35] Hardy A, Casabianca L, Hardy E, Grimaud O, Meyer A. Combined reconstruction of the anterior cruciate ligament associated with anterolateral tenodesis effectively controls the acceleration of the tibia during the pivot shift. Knee Surgery, Sports Traumatology, Arthroscopy. 2017;**25**(4):1117-1124

[36] Sonnery-Cottet B, Thaunat M, Freychet B, Pupim BH, Murphy CG, Claes S. Outcome of a combined anterior cruciate ligament and anterolateral ligament reconstruction technique with a minimum 2-year follow-up. The American Journal of Sports Medicine. 2015;**43**(7):1598-1605

[37] Sonnery-Cottet B, Daggett M, Fayard JM, Ferretti A, Helito CP, Lind M, et al. Anterolateral ligament expert group consensus paper on the management of internal rotation and instability of the anterior cruciate ligament—Deficient knee. Journal of Orthopaedics and Traumatology. 2017;**18**(2):91-106

[38] Wytrykowski K, Swider P, Reina N, Murgier J, Laffosse JM, Chiron P, et al. Cadaveric study comparing the biomechanical properties of grafts used for knee anterolateral ligament reconstruction. Arthroscopy. 2016;**32**(11):2288-2294

[39] Helito CP, Bonadio MB, Gobbi RG, da Mota E Albuquerque RF, Pécora JR, Camanho GL, et al. Combined intra- and extra-articular reconstruction of the anterior cruciate ligament: The reconstruction of the knee anterolateral ligament. Arthroscopy Techniques. 2015;**4**(3):e239-e244

[40] Ferreira MC, Zidan FF, Miduati FB, Fortuna CC, Mizutani BM, Abdalla RJ. Reconstruction of anterior cruciate ligament and anterolateral ligament using interlinked hamstrings—Technical note. Revista Brasileira de Ortopedia. 2016;**51**(4):466-470

[41] Smith JO, Yasen SK, Lord B, Wilson AJ. Combined anterolateral ligament and anatomic anterior cruciate ligament reconstruction of the knee.

Knee Surgery, Sports Traumatology, Arthroscopy. 2015;**23**(11):3151-3156

[42] Wagih AM, Elguindy AM. Percutaneous reconstruction of the anterolateral ligament of the knee with a polyester tape. Arthroscopy Techniques. 2016;**5**(4):e691-e6e7

[43] Chahla J, Menge TJ, Mitchell JJ, Dean CS, LaPrade RF. Anterolateral ligament reconstruction technique: An anatomic-based approach. Arthroscopy Techniques. 2016;**5**(3):e453-e457

[44] Helito CP, Demange MK, Bonadio MB, Tirico LE, Gobbi RG, Pecora JR, et al. Radiographic landmarks for locating the femoral origin and tibial insertion of the knee anterolateral ligament. The American Journal of Sports Medicine. 2014;**42**(10):2356-2362

[45] Saithna A, Thaunat M, Delaloye JR, Ouanezar H, Fayard JM, Sonnery-Cottet B. Combined ACL and anterolateral ligament reconstruction. JBJS Essential Surgical Techniques. 2018;**8**(1):e2

[46] Lutz C, Sonnery-Cottet B, Imbert P, Barbosa NC, Tuteja S, Jaeger JH. Combined anterior and anterolateral stabilization of the knee with the iliotibial band. Arthroscopy Techniques. 2016;**5**(2):e251-e256

[47] Sonnery-Cottet B, Barbosa NC, Tuteja S, Daggett M, Kajetanek C, Thaunat M. Minimally invasive anterolateral ligament reconstruction in the setting of anterior cruciate ligament injury. Arthroscopy Techniques. 2016;**5**(1):e211-e215

[48] Delaloye JR, Murar J, Vieira TD, Saithna A, Barth J, Ouanezar H, et al. Combined anterior cruciate ligament repair and anterolateral ligament reconstruction. Arthroscopy Techniques. 2019;**8**(1):e23-ee9

[49] Ferretti A, Monaco E, Ponzo A, Basiglini L, Iorio R, Caperna L, et al. Combined intra-articular and extra-articular reconstruction in anterior cruciate ligament-deficient knee: 25 years later. Arthroscopy. 2016;**32**(10):2039-2047

[50] Helito CP, Camargo DB, Sobrado MF, Bonadio MB, Giglio PN, Pécora JR, et al. Combined reconstruction of the anterolateral ligament in chronic ACL injuries leads to better clinical outcomes than isolated ACL reconstruction. Knee Surgery, Sports Traumatology, Arthroscopy. 2018;**26**(12):3652-3659

[51] Ferretti A. Extra-articular reconstruction in the anterior cruciate ligament deficient knee: A commentary. Joints. 2014;**2**(1):41-47

[52] Ramaniraka NA, Saunier P, Siegrist O, Pioletti DP. Biomechanical evaluation of intra-articular and extra-articular procedures in anterior cruciate ligament reconstruction: A finite element analysis. Clinical Biomechanics (Bristol, Avon). 2007;**22**(3):336-343

[53] Rezende FC, de Moraes VY, Martimbianco AL, Luzo MV, da Silveira Franciozi CE, Belloti JC. Does combined intra- and extraarticular ACL reconstruction improve function and stability? A meta-analysis. Clinical Orthopaedics and Related Research. 2015;**473**(8):2609-2618

Section 3

Knee Replacement

Chapter 4

Medial Epicondyle Osteotomy for Balancing Severe Varus Knee

Gabriel Stan

Abstract

Varus malalignment is the most common deformity leading to total knee arthroplasty (TKA) for knee arthritis. For correcting this deformity, a stepwise approach is used by surgeons during TKA. When a severe varus malalignment is present, there are some concerns regarding balancing procedure, meaning that aggressive release of medial structures could lead to instability and need for a more constrained implant. In this chapter, the results of an unconventional method for balancing severe varus malalignment are shown. This method is medial epicondyle osteotomy (MEO). For this reason, a total of 135 knees with severe varus deformity were studied. In 65 cases, the MEO technique was used for balancing during TKA. The other 70 cases were balanced using additional resection of medial tibial plateau. Clinical and radiological outcomes were measured before and after surgery for both groups. Also the results were compared to a control group consisting of 50 patients with TKA for varus deformity less than 15 degrees. The amount of resected tibial bone was noted for study groups. Range of motion, the Knee Society Score (KSS), frontal laxity, and correction of femoro-tibial angle were studied. Frontal laxity decreased from $12.81° \pm 3.9°$ to $0.37° \pm 1.2°$ ($P < 0.001$). The results showed no statistically significant differences between groups regarding the KSS, range of motion, femoro-tibial angle, and frontal laxity. The amount of resected tibial bone and the mean thickness of the polyethylene insert were statistically significantly smaller in the MEO group. MEO technique could be useful when treating severe varus arthritis knee during TKA by avoiding aggressive medial release and malalignment. Also the bone stock is preserved.

Keywords: medial epicondyle osteotomy , knee varus deformity, total knee arthroplasty, prosthetic outcomes, survivorship

1. Introduction

Total knee arthroplasty is a common surgical procedure for the end stage of knee arthritis, providing long-term pain relief and patient satisfaction. Although many studies have measured the success of knee arthroplasty in terms of survival, another important aspect of TKA is its functional outcome; that is, postoperatively, patients should be free of pain and able to perform daily activities such as standing, walking, and stair-climbing.

The varus knee is the most common deformity that requires total knee arthroplasty. Malalignment affects articular hyaline cartilage, menisci, subchondral bone, and ligaments, and contributes to progression of osteoarthritis (OA). When varus

 IntechOpen

alignment is present, the forces passing the knee are unequally distributed between condyles with an increased load passing through medial condyle due to an increase of the adduction moment during gait [1].

Anatomical changes are present in varus knee as a result of deforming forces. According to Puthumanapully, some reference axes and surface features are significantly different to normal knees [2]. For the femur, he found less femoral anteversion in varus knees. In the tibia, the tubercle (and tibial tubercle axis) was externally rotated and there was a medial tilt of the tibial plateau in the coronal plane. The coronal slope was found to be significantly more ($P = 0.001$) in varus knees (3.5°) when compared to normal knees (0°), indicating that the slope contributes to the varus deformity. Normal femoral version has been reported to be varied between 10° and 20° [3]. Retroversion or decreasing femoral anteversion is associated with external rotation of the knee and varus deformity contributing to the development of OA in adults [4]. Authors like Bretin and Papaioannou showed that loads shift from center to medial compartment when external femoral malrotation is present [5, 6].

OA also affects the anatomy of superficial medial collateral ligament (MCL), which is the main structure providing medial stability. These changes are secondary to fibrosis of the posteromedial complex, to impingement of marginal osteophytes, and to extrusion of the medial meniscus. According to Haidar, there is no shortening of the MCL in knee OA. There are deforming structures such as the oblique ligament with adhesion and thickening of posteromedial corner structures. Those changes are supposed to cause a posterior bowing to the superficial MCL without an actual shortening of the ligament. The scarring tissue in the posteromedial corner and the adhesion act as a soft phyte tensioning and deform the ligament and the posterior capsule [7].

Ignorance, fear of surgery, access to alternative and traditional medicine, and the high costs of treatment are among main reasons that contribute to late presentation for treatment. Factors like age of the patients, level of activity or disease progression have been discussed when deciding to choose methods of treatment in knee osteoarthritis (OA). Financial aid is a leading factor in decision-making of treating OA. Conservative treatment in knee osteoarthritis is also expensive because it fails to correct the malalignment and abnormal joint loading. The disease will progress and the TKA will be the optimal solution for treatment. Severe preoperative deformities have long been a challenge for surgeons performing total knee arthroplasty.

Limb alignment and proper soft tissue balance are the main factors that influence long-term results of TKA in terms of survivorship. What kind of alignment should be obtained, anatomical, mechanical, or kinematic, is still a matter of debate, but everyone agrees that a balanced prosthetic knee will provide better results. Most of the authors state that the mechanical alignment provides the best chances in terms of survivorship of TKA. Mechanical alignment means that femoral cut is perpendicular to the mechanical axis of the femur and tibial cut is perpendicular to the mechanical axis of the tibia [8].

Technical flows are challenging for surgeons no matter the surgical strategy. A part of this issue is represented by the instruments' errors. The accuracy of obtaining the desired angle of femoral distal cut is dependent on the ability to actually engage the intramedullary rod in the medullary canal respect the anatomic axis of the femor. This maneuver is influenced by the rod length and diameter and the intramedullary diameter of the femoral canal. The location of the entry hole also could have an impact upon alignment. Do to this, the surgeon must be aware that even if he/she is aiming for a mechanical alignment, for example, the instruments and placement of the entry holes could lead to errors. Alignment is critical to load transfer, both at the articular surface and at the implant-host interface, and hence essential for the success of total knee replacement (TKA). Most of the early failures of TKAs are related to technical flaws. Valgus or varus malpositioning of the tibial component of a total knee implant may cause increased propensity for loosening or implant wear and they may eventually lead to revision surgery [9]. Experimental and clinical data indicate that, in order to achieve optimal mid-term and long-term results of a TKR, good alignment in the frontal plane of the lower limb is mandatory.

Releasing the superficial MCL can sometimes lead to a major instability of the knee and other surgical methods should be assessed for balancing the prosthetic knee in cases of severe varus deformity when aggressive MCL release is expected. A severe varus deformity (more than 15 degrees) is a challenge in terms of the type and extent of release required. More constrained types of implants may be needed if the MCL cannot be trusted.

A balanced knee must be the goal of every TKA because this will increase the chances for a better survivorship [10–13]. When malalignment is present, some parts of the soft tissue around the knee are contracted and must be released, thus leading to correction of the deformity [14, 15].

When severe varus deformity is present, medial structures become fibrous. Among the methods used to correct severe varus deformity, the most common are subperiosteal release of the superficial medial collateral ligament and joint line release of the medial collateral ligament. Some other methods like medial epicondyle osteotomy (MEO) and tibial reduction osteotomy are less used due to concerns regarding survivorship [16].

For this study, we used the medial epicondyle osteotomy technique because we believe that this method will allow early recovery, bone stock preservation, and a good overall alignment of the limb as we will show later in this chapter. Some authors also used the MEO technique in the past, but their method involves subsequently reattaching the medial epicondyle with screws, sutures, or anchors in an optimal position for balancing the prosthetic knee, which will not allow early rehabilitation after surgery. We did not reattach this fragment and early rehabilitation program was started. The goal of our study was to underline the results of TKA after using MEO as a balancing method for severe varus deformity. The results were compared with those of TKA after using additional resection of the tibial medial plateau to correct this deformity and to those of TKA for varus deformity less than 15 degrees when standard measures were used for balancing.

2. Materials and methods

Between April 2006 and April 2017, we performed 135 TKAs on patients with severe preoperative varus (of more than 15°). The control group included 50 patients with TKA for preoperative varus less than 15°. In 65 cases (40 female and 25 men), the MEO technique was used, and in 70 cases (45 female and 25 men), additional resection of the tibial medial plateau. The mean age at the time of the TKA in MEO group was 68.6; mean height, 1.72 m; and mean weight, 76 kg. In the resection group, the mean age was 65.4 years; mean height, 1.77 m; and mean weight, 76.9 kg. In the control group, there were 30 female and 20 male patients; mean age was 62.5; mean height was 1.71 m; and mean weight was 76 kg.

Patients with preoperative valgus and secondary OA to trauma or inflammatory diseases were not included in the study. All surgeries were performed by the same main surgeon, using the medial-parapatellar and subvastus approaches. The same type of cemented postero-stabilized knee prosthesis was implanted in all cases (Zimmer Nexgen).

No full weight bearing X Ray films were available for this study, so the distal femoral cut was performed at 5° of valgus relative to the anatomical axis of the femur, using an intramedullary rod. The tibial cut was perpendicular to the tibial mechanical axis, also using an intramedullary guide. A 3° femoral external rotation was set in almost every case. Rotation of the femoral component was decided using Whiteside's line, transepicondylar axis, and posterior condylar reference. A combined anterior and posterior referencing was used for sizing of femur.

All patients underwent stepwise sequential medial soft tissue release consisting of deep MCL, posteromedial release, superficial MCL, and pes anserinus. All the osteophytes were removed. Bony defects were managed with the cement or structural bone grafts and screws. No stem extenders were used. For the control group, no further measures were necessary to balance the prosthetic knee.

For both study groups, these steps were insufficient for balancing the knee and therefore further action was necessary.

In the first group, the surgeon performed a medial epicondyle osteotomy, containing the insertion of the MCL, starting with a saw-blade and finishing with an osteotome (**Figure 1**). Then, a valgus stress was applied lowering the epicondyle to its new position. The inferior margin of the epicondyle was cut with a rongeur for not interfering with the articular part of the implant during movements. No fixation method was used for the epicondyle. The flexion and extension gaps were assessed for balance.

In the second group, as the medial compartment was still tight in extension and flexion, the surgeon performed a secondary asymmetrical tibial coronal recut using the specific instrument and removed an extra 2 mm of bone from the medial tibial plateau (**Figure 2**). Thus proceeding, the extension and flexion gaps were equal and the knee was balanced.

For all cases, the patella was resurfaced and no tourniquet was used. Rehabilitation started immediately after surgery, with alternative positioning of the knee in flexion-extension. On day 1 after surgery, all patients started active motion of the operated knee with flexion-extension exercises. Full weight bearing was allowed form day 1, using no brace for protection. No passive motion device was needed. Postoperative follow-up was scheduled 6 weeks, 3 months, 6 months, and 1 year after the surgery, and once per year afterward. The mean follow-up for the study was 7 years (± 3).

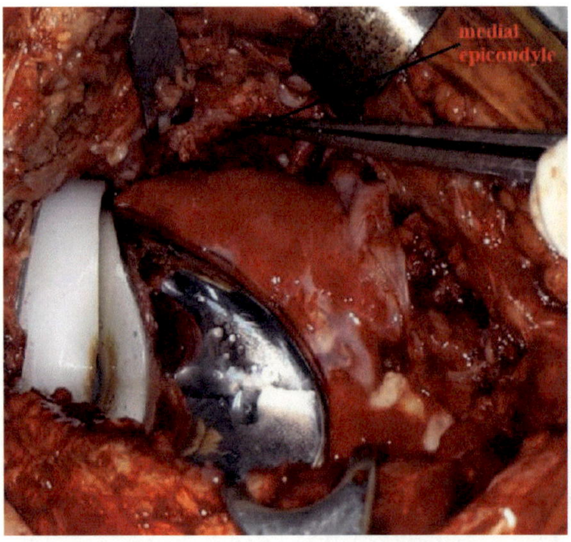

Figure 1.
Medial epicondyle osteotomy with TKA.

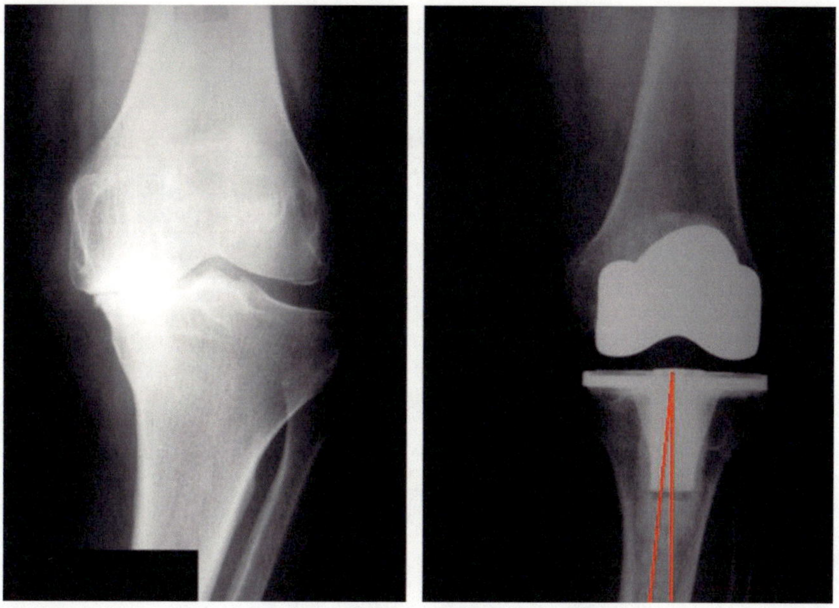

Figure 2.
Additional medial tibial resection (note the varus malposition of tibial component).

The main inclusion criterion for the study group was preoperative varus deformity greater than 15°. The outcomes were measured: Knee Society score (KSS), the range of the motion (ROM), clinical frontal laxity of the knee, femoro-tibial angle, the mean thickness of the polyethylene insert, the amount of resected tibial medial plateau bone, and the union state of the osteotomy site. The amount of resected tibial medial plateau bone was defined as the difference between preoperative and postoperative distance from a perpendicular to the axis of tibia through the peroneal head and a perpendicular to the same axis through the lowermost point of the tibial medial plateau in anteroposterior Rx incidence. The choice of surgical technique was random and we did not use any criteria for performing one or other in this study, but we selected the patients who had a preoperative varus deformity greater than 15°.

Statistical tests were performed using SPSS software. Paired Samples Test was used to compare the results. The 0.05 level was used to denote statistical significance throughout testing.

3. Results

There were no statistically significant differences regarding personal characteristics (age, sex, height, and weight) between the two groups and the control group. No differences were noted regarding postoperative outcomes of KSS, range of motion, femoro-tibial angle, and frontal laxity.

The results are summarized in **Table 1**.

We observed a significant statistical difference regarding positioning of tibial component between groups. The mean angle between tibial component and tibial mechanical axis was 1° ± 3.5°of varus for the MEO group, and 4° ± 2.5° of varus for the resection group ($P < 0.001$). In the control group, the angle was 0.7° ± 2.3°.

The mean thickness of the polyethylene insert was 12.5 ± 1.24 mm in the MEO group and 13.61 ± 1.59 mm in the second group, with statistically significant $P = 0.005$.

Group		KSS	ROM	F-T angle	Frontal laxity
MEO	Preop.	18.15 ± 15.6	72.3° ± 23.5°	25.3° ± 5.51° varus	12.43° ± 3.5°
	Postop.	94.1 ± 5.6	112.3° ± 10.8°	4.0° ± 1.18° valgus	0.32° ± 1.3°
Resection	Preop.	21.44 ± 13.6	86.8° ± 15.5°	24.7° ± 5.1° varus	12.81° ± 3.9°
	Postop.	91.7 ± 7.6	115.4° ± 8.4°	4.1° ± 0.97° valgus	0.37° ± 1.2°
Control	Preop.	25.15 ± 12.1	76.4° ± 24.3°	15.6° ± 7.41° varus	8.81° ± 2.8°
	Postop.	96.3 ± 5.6	118.3° ± 9.7°	2.0° ± 1.2° valgus	1.34° ± 1.2°

Table 1.
Results after TKA for the study groups.

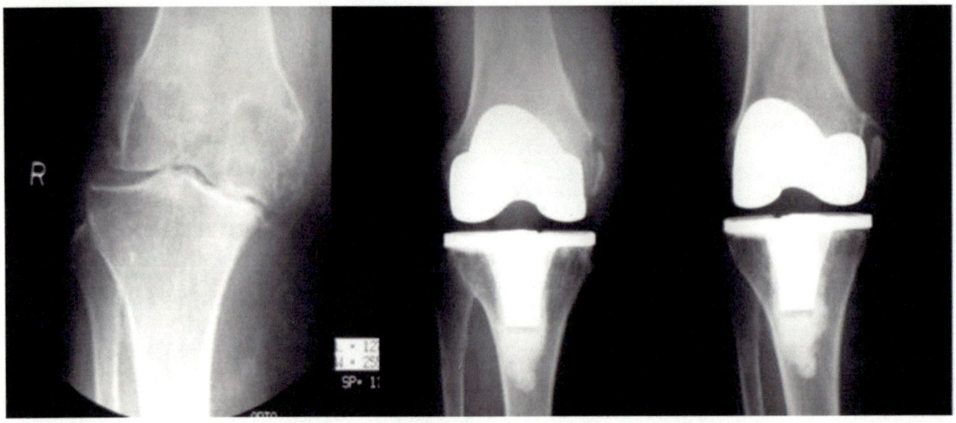

Figure 3.
Medial epicondyle osteotomy Rx (3 months and 5 years follow up).

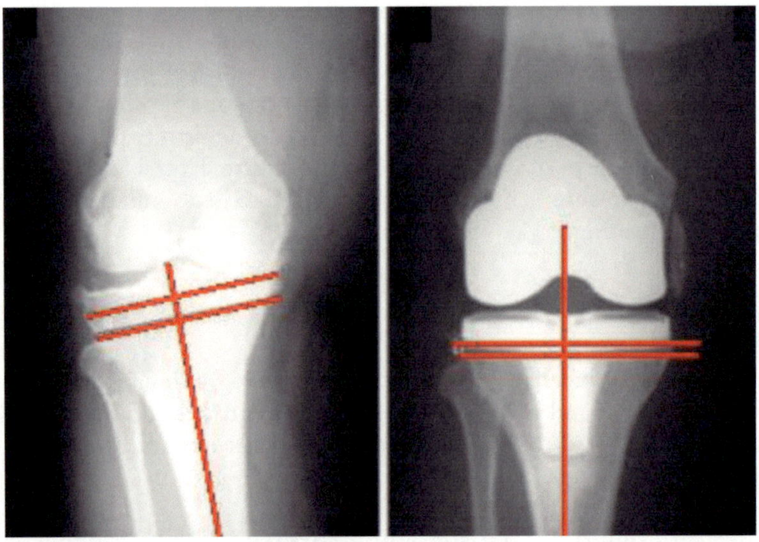

Figure 4.
The amount of tibial medial plateau resected bone- MEO.

For all knees with medial epicondyle osteotomy, a fibrous union occurred at the site of osteotomy (**Figure 3**). In this group, the amount of resected tibial medial plateau bone (**Figures 4** and **5**) was statistically significantly smaller than in the other group (1.33 ± 0.46 mm in the MEO group and 3.73 ± 2.5 mm in the other group; P < 0,001).

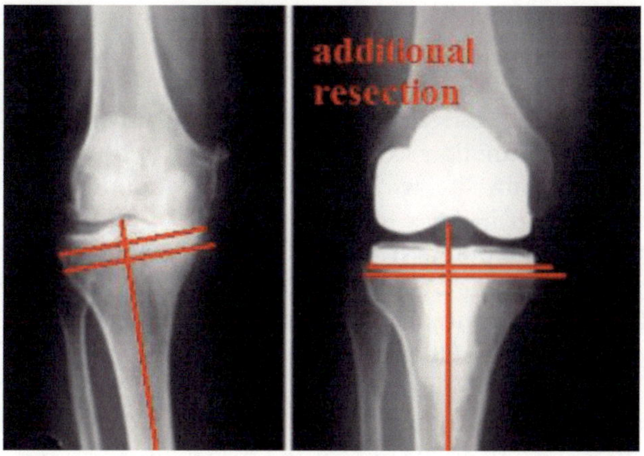

Figure 5.
The amount of tibial medial plateau resected bone (an additional resection of tibial medial plateau case).

Residual frontal laxity was present in four cases, two in the MEO group and two in the second one. No revision surgery was necessary for any of the cases at the last follow-up.

4. Discussion

The varus knee is the most common deformity that requires total knee arthroplasty. Severe varus deformity grossly affects normal anatomy of the knee, meaning that bone and soft tissue are affected by the disease.

For better survivorship of a knee implant, it is mandatory to achieve a proper alignment and a perfect balance of total knee prosthesis. It is a great challenge for surgeons to balance a severe varus knee due to changes in the anatomy of medial compartment. Fibrosis of the posteromedial complex, marginal osteophytes, extrusion of the medial meniscus, adhesion and thickening of the oblique ligament with all the posterior medial complex, and posterior bowing to the superficial MCL are problems that must be corrected during surgery. MCL release is very important in balancing the fixed varus deformity. The surgeon must progressively release the medial soft tissue until it reaches the length of lateral structures. The endpoint of the release is when the knee is stable and the alignment is optimal. In severe varus deformity, the separation of the periosteal layer from the tibia is distal to the MCL attachment. For this reason, some authors raised concerns about the integrity of the MCL after aggressive release. Releasing the superficial MCL can sometimes lead to a major instability of the knee, requiring a more constrained implant [7]. Our method of medial epicondyle osteotomy for severe varus deformity could prevent this problem.

There are few literature reports that describe MEO as a method of balancing the prosthetic knee. Engh has described his results after medial epicondyle osteotomy during TKA. He performed this procedure on 80 patients [16]. The clinical results showed the KSS improvement from 42 to 93 points after surgery and the range of motion increase from 101 to 111 degrees. He has found no instability in his patients group during the follow-up period. Regarding frontal laxity, the mean varus-valgus stability measured 14.2 points (Knee Society scale, 0–15 points). Improvement of function and patient satisfaction was found in 95% of the cases. In every case of his study, the osteotomized epicondyle was fixed during surgery at the optimal position for balance. Despite this, bone union occurred only in 54% of the knees and fibrous union occurred in 46%. No symptoms like tenderness, restricted motion, or other were associated with fibrous union. Other authors like Sim and Kwak reported their results after using medial epicondylar osteotomy for treating varus deformity in 32 cases [17]. Clinical and radiological outcomes, including the Knee Society score (KSS), the function score (FS), the range of the motion (ROM), the union state of the osteotomy site, were measured. They found an improvement of KSS after surgery from 46.5 ± 7.6 to 89.1 ± 5.9 points ($P < 0.001$). The FS increased from 39.5 ± 9.2 to 84.2 ± 8.5 points ($P < 0.001$). Also the range of motion was better after the surgery (101.5° ± 28.2° to 116.0° ± 10.8°; $P = 0.006$). A significant number of patients presented fibrous union on the osteotomy site despite the fixation of the condyle during procedure (10 patients). Bone union occurred only in 22 knees. There was no significant difference regarding clinical outcomes between the bone union group and the fibrous union group ($P = 0.175$). The femoro-tibial angle was corrected from an 8.2° ± 5.0°-varus to a 5.6° ± 1.5°-valgus ($P < 0.001$). Despite the fact that in both studies the epicondyle was fixed with sutures or screws, a major part of the patients presented fibrous union of the epicondyle. The authors concluded that there was no significant difference between the bone union group and the fibrous union group. We do not consider that any reattachment of the epicondyle is necessary, and in consequence, we did not perform fixation in any of the cases. Also no splinting after the surgery was used and the rehab program was started immediately, avoiding knee stiffness and accelerating recovery.

Nobody could tell for sure the ideal positioning of the knee prosthetic components. The disagreement among surgeons is amplified by the significant number of unsatisfied patients with TKA.

Most of the authors state that mechanical alignment provides the best chances in terms of survivorship of TKA. Mechanical alignment means that femoral cut is perpendicular to the mechanical axis of the femur and tibial cut is perpendicular to the mechanical axis of the tibia. If mechanical alignment is achieved, it means that mechanical axis of the leg passes through the center of the knee and the loads are equally distributed between medial and lateral compartments. The native knee interline is inclined about 3 degrees in varus, meaning that the mechanical alignment will change it to 0 degrees, changing the normal anatomy of the knee. The proximal tibial joint line is therefore converted from 87 degrees (3 degrees of varus) to 90 degrees and the distal femoral line from 87 degrees (3 degrees of valgus) to 90 degrees.

For these considerations, some authors proposed the so-called "anatomic alignment" when the tibial component was placed at 3 degrees of varus and the femoral component at 3 degrees of valgus, and overall alignment to be neutral [18]. There is an important variability in natural alignment among population. A significant part of neutral alignment is not normal, leading to distalization of the joint line on the lateral compartment, which can cause anterior knee pain. The concept of restoring constitutional alignment rather than mechanical has gained more interest recently. For the supplementary tibial resection group in our study, we have created the situation of placing the tibial component in varus. In case of a medio-lateral tibial plateau length of 8 cm, an additional resection of 2 mm from medial side lead to a maximum 3 degrees of varus positioning of tibial implant. Attention should be paid in cases where this additional cut adds to a previous unknown error of first cuts due to the instrument's or surgeon's mistake, and this could lead to a supplemental varus, and potential danger in terms of survivorship.

Other authors showed that a femoral component placed in 7° valgus, with tibial plateau placed at 90° to the long axis of the tibia, provides equal force distribution between the medial and lateral plateaus and consecutively best chances for survivorship [19]. According to Howell, kinematically aligning the knee means coaligning the transverse axis of the femoral component with the primary transverse axis in the femur about which the tibia flexes and extends and placing the tibial component so that the longitudinal axis of the tibia is perpendicular to the transverse axis in the femur, about which the tibia flexes and extends [20]. This means that the femoral cut is plus 1°–2° in valgus and tibial cut, plus 1°–2° in varus compared with the mechanically aligned total knee arthroplasty [21]. The authors who propose this approach state that restoring mechanical alignment is unnatural in patients with constitutional varus and valgus alignment and could cause higher strain in collateral ligaments [22]. They say that by restoring the native alignment, patients will have better clinical and functional outcome scores as compared with patients in whom the limb alignment is corrected to neutral [23]. The present general consensus is that overall mechanical femoro-tibial alignment should be 0 ± 3 degrees, thus providing the best survivorship chances for the knee implant [24]. No matter of the technique used for TKA, the next important problem for surgeons are technical flows. The accuracy of obtaining the desired angle of femoral distal cut is dependent on the ability to actually engage the intramedullary rod in the medullary canal to be in line with anatomical axis of the femor. This maneuver is influenced by the rod length and diameter and the intramedullary diameter of the femoral canal. The location of the entry hole also could have an impact upon alignment. Do to this, the surgeon must be aware that even if he/she is aiming for a mechanical alignment, for example, the instruments and placement of the entry holes could lead to errors. Regarding tibial component alignment, we observed a significant difference between groups. For the MEO group, the alignment was neutral (1°± 3.5°) and in the resection group, the alignment was mainly in varus (4° ± 2.5°). In 90% of MEO group cases, the tibial component is placed in line with mechanical axis. Only 5% of the knees from the second group present 90° tibial component placement. The vast majority of them are outliers due to additional asymmetric tibial varus cut. The MEO is a method that increases chances for a mechanical alignment of the prosthetic knee.

5. Conclusion

Based on our results, we suggest that the outcomes of TKA with MEO are similar to those with additional resection of the tibial medial plateau and to those from the control group. No revision surgery was needed at the last follow-up in any of the cases.

Some advantages of medial epicondyle osteotomy have resulted from this study. First of all, it avoids excessive weakening of the medial collateral ligament in cases of severe contracture of medial structures by lowering the epicondyle instead of aggressive releasing of the ligament. This will prevent also the need for a more constrained implant. The exposure during surgery is much easier and avoids complications like extensor mechanism disruption. It is a technique that provides optimal conditions for obtaining neutral overall alignment of the limb, minimizing the risk of malpositioning the tibial component, which is higher in cases of additional tibial resection. The tibial bone loss is less than that in additional resection group which is better for revision surgery.

This study highlights early and mid-term results of TKA with medial epicondyle osteotomy. Further analyses are necessary to assess the long-term results of this technique, especially in terms of survivorship. So far, there are no differences between groups regarding patient satisfaction, range of motion, or survivorship.

Author details

Gabriel Stan
Carol Davila Faculty of Medicine, Elias University Hospital, Bucharest, Romania

*Address all correspondence to: gabisus2000@yahoo.com

References

[1] Amis AA. Biomechanics of high tibial osteotomy. Knee Surgery, Sports Traumatology, Arthroscopy. 2013;**21**:197-205. DOI: 10.1007/s00167-012-2122-3

[2] Puthumanapully PK, Harris SJ, Leong A, Cobb JP, Amis AA, Jeffers J. A morphometric study of normal and varus knees. Knee Surgery, Sports Traumatology, Arthroscopy. 2014;**22**(12):2891-2899. DOI: 10.1007/s00167-014-3337-2

[3] Cibulka MT. Determination and significance of femoral neck anteversion. Physical Therapy. 2004;**84**:550-558

[4] Tönnis D, Heinecke A. Diminished femoral antetorsion syndrome: A cause of pain and osteoarthritis. Journal of Pediatric Orthopedics. 1991;**11**:419-431. DOI: 10.1097/01241398-199107000-00001

[5] Bretin P, O'Loughlin PF, Suero EM, Kendoff D, Ostermeier S, Hüfner T, et al. Influence of femoral malrotation on knee joint alignment and intra-articular contract pressures. Archives of Orthopaedic and Trauma Surgery. 2011;**131**:1115-1120. DOI: 10.1007/s00402-010-1210-4

[6] Papaioannou T, Digas G, Bikos C, Karamoulas V, Magnissalis E. Femoral neck version affects medial femorotibial loading. ISRN Orthopedics. 2013;**2013**: 1-6. DOI: 10.1155/2013/328246

[7] Haidar F, Tarabichi S, Osman A, Elkabbani M, Mohamed T. Understanding the pathological changes of varus knee on MRIcan lead to a better algorithm to balance the knee. Orthopaedic Proceedings. 2019;**101-B**(SUPP_4):85

[8] Insall JN, Binazzi R, Soudry M, Mestriner LA. Total knee arthroplasty. Clinical Orthopaedics and Related Research. 1985;**192**:13

[9] Werner F, Ayers D, Maletsky L. The effect of valgus/varus malalignment on load distribution in total knee replacements. Journal of Biomechanics. 2005;**38**:349-355

[10] W-Dahl A, Robertsson O, Lidgren L. Surgery for knee osteoarthritis in younger patients. Acta Orthopaedica. 2010;**81**(2):161-164

[11] Papachristou G, Plessas S, Sourlas J. Deterioration of longterm results following high tibial osteotomy in patients under 60 years of age. International Orthopaedics. 2006;**30**(5):403-408

[12] Edwards E. The eVect of postoperative collateral ligament laxity in total knee arthroplasty. Clinical Orthopaedics. 1998;**236**:44

[13] Hunt MA, Birmingham TB, Bryant D, et al. Lateral trunk lean explains variation in dynamic knee joint load in patients with medial compartment knee osteoarthritis. Osteoarthritis and Cartilage. 2008;**16**:591-599

[14] Mundermann A, Dyrby CO, Hurwitz DE. Potential strategies to reduce medial compartment loading in patients with knee osteoarthritis of varying severity: Reduced walking speed. Arthritis and Rheumatism. 2004;**50**:1172-1178

[15] Birmingham TB, Hunt MA, Jones IC. Test–retest reliability of the peak knee adduction moment during walking in patients with medial compartment knee osteoarthritis. Arthritis and Rheumatism. 2007;**57**:1012-1017

[16] Engh GA. Medial epicondylar osteotomy: A technique used with

primary and revision total knee arthroplasty to improve surgical exposure and correct varus deformity. Instructional Course Lectures. 1999;**48**:153-156

[17] Sim JA, Kwak JH. Short-term follow-up results of medial epicondylar osteotomy for the varus knee in TKA. Journal of Korean Knee Society. 2009;**21**:194-204

[18] Hungerford DS, Krackow KA. Total joint arthroplasty of the knee. Clinical Orthopaedics and Related Research. 1985;**192**:23

[19] Hsu RW, Himeno S, Coventry MB. Normal axial alignment of the lower extremity and load-bearing distribution at the knee. Clinical Orthopaedics. 1990;**255**:215-227

[20] Howell SM, Roth JD, Hull ML. Kinematic alignment in total knee arthroplasty. Definition, history, principle, surgical technique, and results of an alignment option for TKA. Art. 2014;**1**:44-53

[21] Scott W. Kinematic alignment in total knee arthroplasty. In: Insall & Scott Surgery of the Knee. 5th ed. Vol. 121. Churchill Livingstone; 2012. pp. 1255-1268

[22] Gu Y, Roth JD, Howell SM, Hull ML. How frequently do four methods for mechanically aligning a total knee arthroplasty cause collateral ligament imbalance and change alignment from normal in white patients? Journal of Bone and Joint Surgery. 2014;**96**(12):e101

[23] Vanlommel L, Vanlommel J, Claes S, Bellemans J. Slight undercorrection following total knee arthroplasty results in superior clinical outcomes in varus knees. Knee Surgery, Sports Traumatology, Arthroscopy. 2013;**21**(10):2325-2330

[24] HD1 C, Math KR, Scuderi GR. Polyethylene post failure in posterior stabilized total knee arthroplasty. The Journal of Arthroplasty. 2004;**19**(5):652-657

Chapter 5

Complications after Total Knee Arthroplasty

Muhammet Salih AYAS, Muhammet Kalkışım, Ahmet Köse and Orkun Gül

Abstract

Nowadays, the incidence of knee arthritis increases with the prolongation of human life and the increase in world population. As a result, total knee arthroplasty application rates increased and surgeons gained more experience. There have also been technical advances and total knee arthroplasty operations have been performed using better implants. However, despite these developments, the number and variety of complications are increasing. In addition to performing total knee arthroplasty correctly, it is now becoming more important to recognize complications that may or may develop. Variety of complications after total knee replacement; from minor skin problems to life-threatening complications. In this review article, we aimed to investigate early and late complications during and after total knee replacement surgery.

Keywords: knee, total knee arthroplasty, survival, complications

1. Introduction

Total knee arthroplasty is an effective treatment option which has been applied with increasing rates in recent years with its highly satisfactory results. Recently increased total knee arthroplasty (TKA) procedures increase the number of complications too. In addition to proper patient selection, an accurate surgical technique, early diagnosis, and proper management of complications are required. Complications of TKA have a wide range. Complications vary from small skin problems to mortality. The development of complications may be due to many factors. Some of these are listed below:

- Error in surgical technique.
- Medical error.
- Nurse error.
- Patient non-compliance.
- Trauma.
- Associated comorbid diseases.

Reviewing all the risk factors before surgery and being prepared for the complications that may occur may be lifesaving in TKA, which is currently applied frequently. It is important to recognize, identify, and classify the complications in a timely manner in the correct and effective management of complications. The ambiguity about the complications of TKA in the literature helped identify and classify the complications in a study conducted in 2013 by the knee community [1]. According to this study, 22 complications were described. These are [1]:

- Bleeding
- Wound problems
- Thromboembolism
- Neural deficit
- Vascular issues
- Medial collateral ligament injury
- Instability
- Malalignment
- Stiffness-toughness-contracture
- Deep wound infection
- Fracture
- Extensor mechanism injury
- Patellofemoral dislocation
- Tibiofemoral dislocation
- Bearing surface wear
- Osteolysis
- Implant loosening
- Implant breakage
- Reoperation
- Revision
- Re-hospitalization and mortality [1]

When the complications are examined, it is seen that some of them are simple and easy to overcome with a short-term solution, while some of them can be serious and can go to revision arthroplasty. The number of complications such as implant

Intraoperative	Early postoperative	Late postoperative
Vascular injuries	Bleeding	Instability
Neurological complications	Superficial skin problems	Joint stiffness
Extensor mechanism injury Patellar tendon injury Quadriceps tendon injury Patella fractures	Deep skin problems	Periprosthetic joint infection
	Deep vein thrombosis	Periprosthetic fractures
	Pulmonary embolism	Aseptic loosening
		Osteolysis
Medial collateral ligament injury		Patellofemoral joint problems

Table 1.
Intraoperative, early postoperative, and late postoperative complications.

fracture and polyethylene surface wear has been reduced due to the techniques and innovations in implant materials and designs. In a study, it was shown that the most common cause of revisions in the first 5 years postop was infection, and the reasons for revision in the next 5 years were polyethylene loosening [2]. Complications will be classified as intraoperative, early postoperative, and late postoperative complications (**Table 1**).

2. Intraoperative complications

2.1 Vascular injuries

Although arterial injury during knee replacement is rare, it may have serious results from limb loss to mortality. Arterial injuries can be seen as thromboembolism, direct vascular laceration, pseudoaneurysm, and arteriovenous fistula [3]. The incidence is reported to be 0.03–0.2% in the literature [4].

Vascular injuries may develop due to the thermal effect of cement polymerization, joint manipulations, dislocations, and excessive manipulation [5]. Considering the issue as specific to the total knee arthroplasty, care should be taken against vascular injury during posterior cruciate ligament and posterior capsular release during femoral condylar cutting. Atypical localization of vascular structures due to changes in adhesions and normal anatomy in revision cases increases the risk of vascular injury twice as compared to primary cases [6]. Nowadays, increasing procedures of TKA bring about the possibility of vascular injuries although they are rare. Therefore, it is necessary to take precautions against vascular injuries that may develop, to identify risky patients and to make an early diagnosis. For this, a good anamnesis and physical examination are essential. It is important to examine the presence of hypertension, diabetes, smoking, and vascular claudication. Coldness of the extremities to be operated during physical examination, skin atrophy and thinning, prominent vascular structures, ulcerative wound, and distal arterial pulse weakness are the findings that need attention. In addition to these findings, the presence of vascular calcifications in radiological scanning, a history of bypass, and an ankle-brachial index below 0.9 are other findings that should be considered. No tourniquet should be used in patients with the abovementioned conditions [7]. Embolism and arterial insufficiency may develop due to tourniquet effect in patients with vascular disease and atheroma plaque in the superficial artery [8]. It has been shown that during the manipulation of the superficial femoral artery fixed during tourniquet effect, intimal damage may occur [9]. Improper placement of retractors can also cause damage by direct mechanical trauma [10]. Particularly during insertion of the posterior retractor, a 1 cm area in the lateral portion of the midline was identified as a risky area [11]. In a cadaver study, neurovascular structures on the tibial side were mapped on a clock diagram. Accordingly, the popliteal vein at 12 o'clock, the popliteal artery at 1 o'clock, and the anterior tibial artery at 2 o'clock for the left knee were shown as in place [12]. Cautious use of the saw between 11 and 3 o'clock defined in the tibial cutting is important in protecting vascular structures [12].

If vascular injury is suspected the tourniquet should be deflated, and bleeding control should be performed before the incision is closed. The possibility of arterial injury should be taken into consideration in the presence of excessive and pulsatile bleeding and in the absence of peripheral pulses. Although recent studies suggest bleeding control after routine tourniquet deflation prior to incision, its benefit is controversial [13]. The surgeon should perform a postoperative peripheral pulse examination routinely, suspect acute ischemia in the presence of cold and delayed distal capillary filling, and request cardiovascular consultation [14]. Acute ischemia cases with delayed diagnosis of 4–6 hours cause irreversible damage. Prophylactic fasciotomy is performed after revascularization [14].

Pseudoaneurysm may present with pulsatile swelling in the popliteal fossa due to direct damage to the popliteal artery during surgery. Doppler ultrasonography is useful in the diagnosis. In the treatment, excision of the lesion and repair with vascular graft is applied after embolization [15]. Arteriovenous fistula is less common. It usually occurs due to injury to the medial and lateral geniculate arteries and its branches. It may present with pulsatile swelling in the popliteal region that gives "trill." Hemarthrosis or pseudoaneurysm may develop. Ultrasound and angiography are used for diagnosis [16]. The detected lesions should be evaluated together with cardiovascular surgery, and treatment should be planned. Embolization, lesion excision, and graft repair are treatment options [15].

2.2 Neurologic complications

Nerve injuries are rare during TKA. Peroneal nerve injury is the most common of these [17]. Sacral plexopathy and sciatica neuropathy are also seen, although rarely [18]. Risk factors for neurological injury are [19]:

- Flexion deformity
- Advanced valgus deformity
- Presence of an intra-articular hematoma

It has been shown that the risk of nerve injury is increased in patients with rheumatoid arthritis [20]. However, none of these risk factors is directly related to nerve injury [18]. Nerve injury is associated not only with the surgical procedure but also with the anesthesiologist-induced regional anesthesia [21]. Hypertension, diabetes, nerve compression history, presence of tethered cord, and rheumatoid arthritis in the patients increase the risk of neural complications secondary to regional anesthesia [22]. The duration of tourniquet use was associated with nerve injuries. According to this, in the tourniquet applications exceeding 2 hours, the risk of peroneal and tibial nerve injuries including 89% peroneal nerve was determined as 7%. All of these have been shown to get recovery. In procedures exceeding 2 hours, the 10–30-minute break and deflation of the tourniquet reduces the complication rate [19]. Although there is a minimal effect on the functional results of the patients effect on the functional results of the patients during the follow-up, paresthesia and numbness are seen in the distal and lateral site of incision due to the injury of the infrapatellar branch of the saphenous nerve. It is seen in the literature at a rate of 25–76%, and most of these recover spontaneously [23]. Nerve injuries are difficult to detect intraoperatively. In the presence of postoperative nerve injury, physical therapy should be planned immediately. EMG examination is recommended after 3 months [20]. If no improvement is observed, nerve exploration may be planned in the future.

2.3 Extensor mechanism injuries

The extensor mechanism in the knee joint consists of quadriceps muscle group, quadriceps tendon, patella, patellar retinaculum, patellar tendon, and tuberositas tibia. Extensor mechanism integrity may be impaired during surgery [20]. Although extensor mechanism injuries occur more frequently postoperatively, they may also occur intraoperative. The incidence is reported to be between 1 and 12% [24]. The treatment of extensor mechanism injuries is quite difficult and the results are not satisfactory.

2.3.1 Patellar tendon rupture

Rupture usually occurs at the site of insertion to the tuberositas tibia. The risk of development is less than 1% [25]. Less frequently, intratendinous and infrapatellar tendon rupture may also occur [25]. The risk of injury increases when patellar tendon mobility decreases. These are [26]:

- Patella baja
- Previous surgery
- Severe limitation of movement in the knee

The risk of tendon injury especially on stiffness knees due to forced manipulations and during the tibial bone cutting increases during surgery. The most common injury mechanism after surgery is falling onto the knee while knee is flexed [27]. Patellar tendon injury without trauma is seen by weakening the tendon after repeated contact of the polyethylene insert [27].

In patients with patellar tendon rupture, pain, swelling, loss of extension, and a palpable defect at the infrapatellar side are detected.

Age, functional status, tendon rupture localization, and soft tissue status are the determinants of the treatment. Splitting and bracing are considered in patients who do not have functional expectations and are unsuitable for surgery [28]. Treatment of acute patellar tendon rupture intraoperative is primary repair [26]. Several techniques have been described using staple and suture anchors for this purpose [28]. Reconstruction techniques are used in patients with poor soft tissue quality. For this purpose, biological materials (hamstring tendon autograft, achilles, peroneal tendon autograft, and extensor mechanism allograft) and synthetic materials can be used [28–30].

2.3.2 Quadriceps tendon rupture

It is very rare. It is especially seen as a rupture from the intersion side to the patella. Excessive patella cutting, previous quadriceps snip, or V-Y tipping are risk factors [28]. The clinical finding is similar to patellar tendon rupture.

Good results have been reported with plaster cast in partial tears [31]. Extensor loss greater than 20° is considered a complete tear and should be treated surgically.

It has unsatisfactory results due to high complication rates and tendency to re-rupture depending on tendon quality and soft tissue condition.

2.3.3 Patella fractures

Patellar fractures are the most common injury among the extensor mechanism injuries [24, 32]. In general, the risk increases with excessive bone cutting while preparing for patellar component. Patellar fracture may occur by direct trauma to the anterior knee or as an avulsion due to the pull of the quadriceps muscle [32].

For diagnosis, pain, swelling, and extensor insufficiency are detected in front of the knee. Lateral knee radiography and tomography in case of clinical suspicion are helpful imaging methods for the diagnosis.

A classification has been developed to assess implant stability and extensor mechanism continuity for periprosthetic patella fractures [33]. Type 1, a stable implant and continuous extensor mechanism; Type 2, a stable implant but a discontinuous extensor mechanism; and Type 3, which indicates instable implant and discontinuous extensor mechanism. Patellar bone stock is classified as 3A if good and 3B if poor. Treatment is also determined according to this classification. Conservative treatment methods are preferred for type 1 cases, while surgical treatments are preferred for types 2 and 3 [33]. In recent studies, it is reported that 40–50% of complications occur and more than half strength loss of extensor mechanism is observed [34].

2.4 Medial collateral ligament injury

During total knee replacement, medial collateral ligament (MCL) is important for soft tissue stabilization and coronal plan stability. The incidence of iatrogenic MCL injury is 2.2–2.7% [35]. In the case of surgical injuries, direct repair, constrained prosthesis use, and even revision at the same session are among the options [36]. Unrecognized MCL injuries during surgery cause early instability. This leads to early implant wear and consequently the need for early revision. Therefore, it is important to diagnose and repair the injury during surgery [37]. Sudden instability in the valgus stress test during knee stabilization indicates MCL injury. Injury may occur from femoral insertion, within the tendon or tibial insertion [38]. Primary repair technique varies according to injury level. Fixation with screw is recommended if MCL injury occurs from its femoral insertion site. Otherwise, if it is through tendon, repairing with insoluble suture technique is recommended. Finally, if MCL injury occurs from its tibial insertion site, both insoluble suture anchor technique and fixation with staple technic are recommended [39, 40]. Factors that increase the risk of medial collateral ligament injury during surgery are as follows [39]:

- Using a larger saw blade than femoral condyle
- Delayed excision of medial side osteophytes
- Performing challenging manipulations of varus-valgus
- Patients with flexion contractures [39]

Patient-related risk factors include obesity and severe deformities [41, 42].

A certain algorithm has not yet been established for the treatment of iatrogenic MCL injuries that occur intraoperative. Many treatment methods with disadvantages and advantages have been used [39, 43, 44]. The traditional method is using constrained prosthesis. However, in this method, it was shown that the stress load on the implant increased and direct repair and treatment with non-constrained prosthesis were recommended instead. In addition, augmentation or increase in polyethylene thickness has been proposed [45]. In one study, it was shown that the risk of instability was 57% in the use of non-constrained prostheses independent of the repair technique after MCL injury [37]. In a 2016 study, four treatment modalities were compared after MCL injury. These are the use of non-constrained prosthesis only, the use of non-constrained prosthesis with primary repair, the use of non-constrained prosthesis only, and the use of constrained prosthesis with primary repair. In 23 patients, the most appropriate treatment method according to the knee community scoring was found to be the use of constrained prosthesis only [46]. However, due to the small number of patients, larger series of studies are needed to determine which treatment is most appropriate.

3. Early postoperative complications

3.1 Bleeding

Bleeding is seen in varying rates between 0 and 39% after TKA [47]. This naturally increases the need for blood transfusion. Intraoperatively, care should be taken about bleeding and good bleeding control is established. Thus, the amount of bleeding is reduced to a minimum. As a result, the risks of immunological reaction due to transfusion are reduced.

Bleeding tolerance is low in patients with comorbid disease and in patients with insufficient cardiac capacity, and the risk of complications increases even in small amounts of bleeding. Preoperative blood preparation before surgery and limitation of the use of anticoagulants are among the measures that can be taken. Precautions during and after TKA surgery can reduce the amount of bleeding. These methods are as follows:

- Use of femoral intramedullary plugs [48]
- Hypotensive anesthesia [49]
- Cryotherapy and Jones bandage [50]
- Use of fibrin tissue adhesive [50, 51]
- Clamping the drain [52–54]
- Application of tranexamic acid [55]

Fibrinolysis is activated by surgical trauma and tourniquet use [56]. Increased fibrinolytic activity causes increased bleeding during TKA. Tranexamic acid shows an anti-fibrinolytic effect by inhibiting the conversion of plasmin to plasminogen [57]. Tranexamic acid can be administered in four different ways: intravenous, oral, intramuscular, and intra-articular [55]. Transition to maximum plasma levels is 30 minutes for intramuscular use, 5–15 minutes for intravenous use, and 2 hours after oral use [58]. Patients with total knee arthroplasty may be treated with a fast-acting intravenous route. Many studies have shown that administration of tranexamic acid after tourniquet deflation and postoperative dose repeat reduces the amount of bleeding and the need for transfusion [59–61]. However, many different protocols for the use of tranexamic acid have been implemented. Preoperative single dose and repeated dose every 8 hours for 3 days have been described in the literature and shown to be effective [62]. In a study conducted in 2011, tranexamic acid was administered at a dose of 10 mg/kg 10 minutes before the tourniquet was opened, and the same dose was repeated 3 hours postoperatively. Five hundred mg tranexamic acid was administered orally 3 times a day for 5 days. At the end of this study, it was shown that the amount of hemorrhage and the rate of transfusion decreased effectively [55].

3.2 Skin healing problems: superficial and deep infections

The incidence of wound problems after TKA is 1–25% [63]. The skin problems may be delayed wound healing, skin necrosis, traumatic or atraumatic separation of the lips of the wound, prolonged serous discharge at the wound site, formation of superficial or deep hematoma, allergic reaction to patch, suture material or dressing materials, bullae formation, fat necrosis, bleeding, keloid formation, and superficial or deep infection [64].

Etiologic reasons that may develop the problem before TKA should be determined in advance, and appropriate measures should be taken [65]. Presence of systemic diseases such as diabetes, hypertension, rheumatoid arthritis, and vascular insufficiency, which may adversely affect wound healing before TKA, should be questioned. Since the soft tissues around the knee are thinner than the other parts of the body, even the smallest problem that may occur at the wound site can cause serious complications. Incision planning should be made carefully in the case of a history of operation from the same place and scarring beforehand, and if necessary, plastic surgery assistance should be taken.

3.2.1 Skin healing problems

Factors adversely affecting wound healing are obesity, hypertension, diabetes, smoking, chronic drug use, steroid use, previous radiotherapy, scarring, inflammatory disease, malnutrition, albumin levels below 3.5 g/dl, and hemoglobin levels below 10 g/dl. Transferrin and lymphocyte levels may also contribute to wound healing problems [66]. Therefore, a detailed anamnesis and physical examination and laboratory examination before surgery give an idea about possible skin problems. Accordingly, measures are taken, replacement therapies are given, and surgery may be postponed until the current pathology is corrected, if necessary. Adjustment of fasting blood sugar levels below 200 g/dl and keeping HbA1C below 6.5 in patients with diabetes will reduce the risk of possible wound problems [67].

Patients with a body mass index above 30 kg/m^2 are 6 times more likely to have infection and wound problems [66]. In obese patients, dietician support should be given before surgery; unnecessary exclusion should be avoided during surgery, and soft tissue surgery should be applied carefully.

A study of smoking patients showed that there were 2 times more wound problems [65]. Because of the vasoconstrictor effect of nicotine in the cigarette, it is recommended to quit smoking 60 days before surgery due to decreased blood supply at the wound site.

Incision planning should be performed in the presence of scar after previous surgery. In the presence of a single longitudinal incision without problems, the same incision should be used. If the old incision cannot be used, a distance of at least 7–8 cm should be left. If there is more than one old incision scar in the anterior part of the knee, the most lateral scar is used considering that the anterior knee feeding is from the medial perforating artery. In addition, the lateral soft tissue flap should not be dissected too much [65]. Unnecessary retractors and additional soft tissue damage should be avoided during surgery. The wound lips should be exactly opposite to each other. Overstretched closing should be avoided. This should be checked with capillary filling time.

Especially in patients with risk factors, it should be performed without tourniquet or at low pressures [65]. Difficult rehabilitation in the early postoperative period should be postponed if possible until it is ensured that there are no wound problems.

Hematoma formation increases the risk of infection [65]. Therefore, measures should be taken to prevent the formation of hematoma. These include no dead space during wound closure, good bleeding control, use of a Jones bandage, and avoidance of overdose of the prophylactic anticoagulants used [65, 68]. Once the hematoma has developed, a needle aspiration can be performed. However, if the hematoma is organized and the drainage cannot be achieved, discharge and debridement can be achieved by arthrotomy under operating room conditions.

The presence of necrosis in the wound leads to catastrophic consequences. Respect to soft tissue is the most important step to prevent necrosis development. The depth of necrosis is important. Superficial necrosis can be treated by local intervention. If larger, debridement and full-thickness skin grafts or fasciocutaneous flaps are required [69]. If necrosis includes full-thickness soft tissue, closure with fascial skin or muscular skin graft should be performed after urgent aggressive debridement [70].

3.2.2 Superficial and deep infections

Despite all current precautions, surgical site infections remain the most serious and feared complications of TKA. After TKA, patients should be followed up with daily dressings, and wound discharge should be evaluated carefully. Prolonged wound discharge is defined as a discharge that lasts more than 48 hours regardless of the amount of drainage [64]. Wet wounds greater than 2×2 cm are considered abnormal after 72 hours and are associated with fat necrosis, hematoma, necrosis, or poor closure of the fascia. They are reported as 1–10% after primary knee replacement [65]. In the early stage of treatment, usually dressing and immobilization for 3–5 days is recommended [71]. Continuous discharge for 72 hours is dangerous. If it exceeds 5 days, debridement should be applied in operating room conditions as it will increase the risk of superficial or deep infection [64].

Superficial infection: It is defined as infection of the soft tissue above the skin—subcutaneous and deep fascia that has not passed under the deep fascia, not opened into the joint cavity. It occurs most frequently in the first 30 days after surgery. The incidence of superficial infection after TKA has been reported as 10% [72]. It may occur through direct contamination or blood. Improper preparation of direct contamination sterilization environment, inadequate surgical field preparation, presence of sloppy surgical team, non-sterile dressing materials, and application may occur as a result of the presence of infected patients in the same environment [73]. The risk of direct contamination can be minimized by precautions. Hematogen contamination can occur if there is any other focus of infection in the body. Therefore, in the presence of a possible infection focus with detailed anamnesis and examination before the operation, the current focus treatment can be planned through detailed examination.

Infection after TKA can be evaluated as patient-related risk factors, surgical intervention-related factors, and postoperative factors [66, 68, 74–77].

- *Patient-related risk factors* include advanced age, previous knee surgery, previous knee infection, steroid use, presence of inflammatory disease, obesity, diabetes, smoking, intravenous drug use, hematologic diseases, oncologic diseases, above ASA score 2, immunosuppressive use, regional skin problems, old incision scars, previous radiotherapy procedures, malnutrition, vascular insufficiency, albumin level below 3.5 g/dl, transferrin level below 200 mg/dl, hemoglobin level below 10 g/dl [78, 79].

- *Surgical intervention related risk factors* include prolonged surgical time of more than 2 hours, absence of laminar flow in the operating room, transfusion, use of hinged knee prosthesis, failure of surgical team to comply with asepsis, and sterility rules [80].

- *Operative period related risk factors* include prolonged hospital stay pre- and postoperative, lack of appropriate antibiotic prophylaxis, hematoma formation, and prolonged wound drainage for more than 5 days [81].

Superficial wound infection is considered with the presence of at least one of the following: discharge from the wound incision, culture of the wound from aseptic conditions, suspicion of infection in clinical evaluation, disproportionate pain, increased temperature, erythema, and localized swelling [79].

In superficial wound infection, unlike deep infection, there is no progressive change in erythrocyte sedimentation rate, C-reactive protein level, and peripheral leukocyte count; the increase is below 25% [82]. In addition, leukocytes in synovial fluid are detected less than 2000/ml, and polymorphonuclear leukocytes are detected under 50%. Alpha defensin and leukocyte esterase tests are negative [71].

When superficial wound infection is detected, the development of deep infection can be prevented by early intervention. Otherwise, it may develop into periprosthetic infection and cause catastrophic results. In the presence of superficial infection, local wound care due to the underlying cause and debridement should be performed if appropriate anti-therapy is required [80]. In the selection of antibiotics, consultation with infectious diseases should be requested. Antibiotherapy is continued after reproduction. If deep infection is excluded in surgical debridement, the joint should not be opened, and the implant should not be touched [83]. Hyperbaric oxygen therapy has a positive effect on appropriate patient selection [84].

3.3 Deep vein thrombosis and pulmonary embolism

Deep vein thrombosis is the general name of thrombosis in the venous circulatory system. It occurs most commonly in the deep veins of the lower extremity [85]. From asymptomatic deep vein thrombosis to pulmonary embolism, which can be fatal, it can be confused with clinical manifestations of varying degrees [85]. It is one of the important complications that increase morbidity and mortality after TKA [86]. Even with mechanical or pharmacological methods, the incidence of asymptomatic DVT is 5.1%, and the incidence of symptomatic DVT is 0.4% [87]. The mortality rate due to pulmonary embolism after TKA is 0.08% [88].

It is important to understand the Virchow triad in the pathogenesis of DVT development. There is a slowdown in blood flow (stasis), endothelial damage, and hypercoagulability [89]. The admixture of fat and bone marrow particles into the venous system after engraving of the femoral canal during TKA explains the hypercoagulability branch of the Virchow triad. Hyperflexion of the leg during surgery and anterior manipulation of the tibia with retractors explain endothelial damage. In addition, this manipulation causes obstruction of the popliteal veins and prolonged immobilization of the leg, leading to venous pooling and stasis [89].

3.3.1 Risk factors

- VTE risk increases after age of 40 and doubles every 10 years after that age [90]. Age increases the risk of VTE regardless of other risk factors.
- Genetic factors are also an important parameter that increases the risk of DVT. Factor V Leiden mutation that causes thrombophilia, as well as protein C, protein S, and antithrombin III deficiency are among the factors that increase the risk of DVT.
- Although tourniquet use has been reported to cause venous stasis, it has been shown that it does not significantly increase the risk of DVT because of its fibrinolytic effect [91, 92].
- The type of anesthesia also affects the risk of developing DVT. General anesthesia has been shown to increase the risk of DVT compared to neuraxial anesthesia (spinal or epidural). Neuroaxial blockade causes vasodilatation in the lower extremities and reduces venous pooling; therefore it explains the mechanism of action [93].
- Other risk factors that increase the risk of DVT are immobilization, smoking, oral contraceptive and hormone use, history of VTE, obesity, malignancy, and difficult knee manipulations.

3.3.2 Diagnosis

A painful, swollen, and reddened leg after TKA should suggest the possibility of DVT. Incomplete DVTs usually do not show signs. Incomplete DVTs are seen especially after arthroplasty. Clinical findings are seen in 1% of all DVT cases. Physical examination findings include redness, swelling, and Homan's sign test and Pratt test positivity. Clinical Wells risk score was established for the diagnosis of deep vein thrombosis [94]. Clinical Wells Scoring criteria are malignancy, paralysis (paresthesia or splinting lower extremity), immobilization for more than 3 days, localized tenderness in the deep venous system, swelling of the lower extremity, 3-cm-diameter differentiation from the other leg, pretibial gode positive edema, history of deep vein thrombosis, and collateral superficial veins. The presence of each risk factor was evaluated as 1 point, and clinical scoring of 3 and above was found to be a high risk for the development of deep vein thrombosis.

Clinical data are not sufficient for the diagnosis of DVT. Therefore, further examination with clinical risk scoring, D-dimer level, Doppler ultrasonography, contrast-enhanced venography, CT, and MRI should be performed. Venography is the best method for the diagnosis of DVT in the lower extremities. The accuracy rate was 97% in the lower extremity veins and 70% in the iliac veins [95]. Venography is not preferred as first-line imaging because it has a 3% risk of DVT and is an invasive method, and also it requires contrast matter that can be toxic to the kidneys. Doppler USG is the most commonly used first-line imaging method because of its cheapness, reproducibility, and patient comfort in the suspicion of DVT. Proximal DVT sensitivity was 96%, distal DVT sensitivity was 44%, and DVT specificity was 93% [96].

Pulmonary embolism should be suspected in the case of sudden shortness of breath, tachypnea, tachycardia, and chest pain after TKA. However, since there are many other diseases with these findings, risk factor assessment and effective differential diagnosis should be made. Wells pulmonary embolism clinical probability scoring was established [97]. Pulmonary angiography is the gold standard for the diagnosis of pulmonary embolism [85].

3.3.3 Prophylaxis

Primary treatment of DVT and related pulmonary embolism is very difficult and cost-effective. Therefore, it is more plausible to establish protocols that prevent the development of DVT and to give ideal prophylaxis. Many pharmacological and mechanical prophylaxis methods are available. The aim is to prevent the development of DVT and not to increase bleeding. Therefore the drug or method of choice should be patient-specific:

- *Mechanical prophylaxis*: The aim is to reduce venous stasis by compressing the lower extremity and to increase fibrinolysis. The risk of hemorrhage is very low, and, if applied correctly, there are almost no complications. Patient compliance is important in mechanical prophylaxis and is the only negative aspect of the method. Mechanical prophylaxis methods include early mobilization, in-bed exercise, use of antithromboembolic socks, and pneumatic compression devices. It has ben shown that intermittent pneumatic compression devices provide as effective prophylaxis as chemical prophylactic agents, and the American College of Chest Physicians (ACCP) recommends the use of mechanical prophylaxis [98].

- *Chemical prophylaxis*: Many agents are used. They all have their own advantages and disadvantages. Risk factors are determined by patient-based evaluation and the most appropriate agent should be preferred:

    - *K vitamin antagonist warfarin*: It prevents the formation of fibrin by inactivating 2, 7, 9, and 10 of the clotting factors. It also inhibits the activation of fibrinolysis-causing protein C and S. Since this effect occurs earlier, it creates a temporary clotting condition. Patients with warfarin should therefore be heparinized until the effect on coagulation factors begins. The anticoagulant effects of warfarin are reversible and monitored by the international normalization rate (INR) measurement. Interaction with other drugs, narrow confidence interval, and dual effect have recently reduced the usage of post-TKA [99, 100].

    - *Heparin*: It acts by inactivating circulating antithrombin III. Antithrombin III also inactivates circulating factors 2, 9, 10, 11, and 12. The use of standard heparin has recently been restricted due to the low risk of bleeding due to low-molecular-weight heparin.

    - *Acetylsalicylic acid*: It acts as an anticoagulant by blocking thromboxane A2, which is necessary for platelet aggression. Recent studies have shown that VTE can be used prophylactically [101].

    - Other oral anticoagulants that may be used: *rivaroxaban (direct factor Xa inhibitor), apixaban (direct factor Xa inhibitor), and dabigatran (direct thrombin inhibitor)*.

4. Late postoperative complications

4.1 Instability

The development of instability after TKA is the third most common cause of revision (17%) after aseptic loosening and infection [102]. Patients present with signs of pain and swelling with movement and weight loss. There may also be pain, emptiness, or abnormal friction and rattling noise in some range of motion.

On the knee during walking, varus or valgus orientation and recurvatum can be seen. Anterior knee pain during sitting up is typical in flexion instabilities. The heaviest table is knee dislocation. The treatment of instability is revision surgery. However, the rate of recurrent instability after revision was 18–60% [103]. This high rate is usually due to the lack of correct identification of the cause of instability.

A clinical classification of knee instability was established. Components of this classification are flexion-extension gap mismatch, component alignment problem, isolated ligament failure, extensor mechanism failure, component loosening, and global instability [103].

4.1.1 Risk factors

The success of total knee replacement depends on the correct alignment of the lower limb mechanical axis. It is recommended that the postoperative lower limb mechanical axis should be in neutral alignment. The tibial cut surface in the coronal plane should be made perpendicular to the mechanical axis of the tibia. Similarly the femoral cut in the coronal plane should be made perpendicular to the mechanical axis of the femur. It is necessary for a stable knee to obtain a rectangular gap in both flexion and extension after bone incisions and soft tissue release in TKA. Balancing the gaps is important to ensure stability and for full range of motion. Flexion gap controlled by posterior femoral condylar cut and tibial cut. Extansion gap controlled by distal femoral condylar cut and the tibial cut. If there is a symmetric gap problem, tibial bone cut is adjusted first; otherwise if there is asymmetric gap problem, adjust femoral bone cut first. For example, if the knee is tight both in extension and flexion, it is called symmetrical gap problem, and its solution is to cut more proximal tibia. The asymmetric gap is one of the most common causes of instability. In some patients, the underlying cause increases the risk of instability. These reasons can be listed as follows:

- Knee with advanced deformity.
- Regional muscle weakness.
- Neuromuscular disease.
- Internal side ligament or posterior cruciate ligament failure.
- Obesity and rheumatoid arthritis.
- Charcot arthropathy

4.1.2 Treatment

It is necessary for a stable knee to obtain a rectangular gap in both flexion and extension after bone incisions and soft tissue release in TKA. If the cavity is larger than the prosthesis, the term symmetrical discrepancy is used. The reason for this instability is that the distal femoral incision or the tibial incision is more than necessary [85].

If the tibial incision is excessive, both extension and flexion will be loose. If this condition is noticed intraoperatively, it is thought that the problem is solved with a thicker insert, but in fact, both the patellofemoral joint problems can arise as the joint line will go down more inferiorly and the early relaxation and fixation problems can arise because the tibial component will sit on the narrower surface.

If the distal femoral incision is excessive, there will be looseness in the extension range. The use of a thick insert during surgery will improve the looseness of the extension, but there will be tightness in flexion [104]. In addition, as the joint line will increase, both the effective distance of collateral ligament will decrease, and patellofemoral joint problems will occur. Therefore, if the distal femoral incision is excessive, the use of distal femoral augment should be preferred instead of the use of a thick insert [105].

Asymmetric mismatches occur when the joint space is trapezoidal rather than rectangular. It occurs mostly during surgery after excessive loosening of the soft tissue and is most commonly seen in extension. In this case, the transition to the restrictive prosthesis should be considered [106].

4.2 Joint stiffness

One of the reasons that greatly affect patient satisfaction after TKA operations is the amount of joint range of motion. To achieve good results, a flexion range of at least 90° is required. Sixty-five degrees of flexion is required during walking; 106° of flexion is required when sitting on a chair and tying shoes. Postoperative limited and painful joint movements significantly reduce patient comfort. A flexion range of less than 90° for 6 weeks after TKA surgery is defined as a rigid knee [107].

4.2.1 Risk factors and causes

Hip osteoarthritis, heterotropic ossification, and reflex symptomatic dystrophy can be considered as independent factors. Inadequate posterior femoral incision and inadequate medial collateral ligament releasing of the knee with severe varus deformity may be among the causes for a rigid knee due to surgical technique [108, 109]. In one study, it was observed that joint stiffness occurred more frequently than unilateral knee arthroplasty in patients who underwent bilateral total knee arthroplasty in the same session, and manipulation was required under anesthesia [110].

Excessive tight extension and flexion gap, tight PCL, malrotation of components, and inadequate tibial slop angle may lead to joint stiffness [108].

One of the most important indicators of joint stiffness is the extremely limited range of motion in the knee before surgery [109]. The range of motion obtained within the surgery should be considered in the determination of joint stiffness. A sudden loss of motion should suggest a mechanical problem, loosening, and infection.

Arthrofibrosis is the most treatment-resistant cause of joint stiffness. It develops due to excessive increase of fibrous tissue in the joint [108].

4.2.2 Treatment

The strongest determinant of postoperative flexion movements is the degree of preoperative flexion. Other than that, age, preoperative diagnosis, and severity of deformity are other factors [111].

The efficacy of conservative treatment is limited in joint stiffness after TKA. Aggressive range of motion improvement of 3.1° was observed with aggressive physical therapy for almost 1 year [112]. It has been shown that the use of continuous passive motion device (CPM) in the early postoperative period reduces bleeding and is beneficial in preventing joint stiffness by reducing the formation of fibrosis [113].

Although there is no consensus in the literature, manipulation under anesthesia should be performed in cases where knee flexion is below 90° between 2 weeks and 3 months. Revision rates are lower in patients with early manipulation [114]. Manipulation is performed under general anesthesia using a muscle relaxant until the knee and hip reach at least 90°. After this procedure, an average gain of 30–47° was reported [115].

If the joint movement limitation continues despite these methods, surgical procedures are performed. These are arthroscopic release, open release and limited revision knee arthroplasty, and total revision knee arthroplasty [116].

4.3 Periprosthetic joint infections

Deep infection after TKA is the most common cause of revision. Systemic complications such as septicemia and cardiopulmonary insufficiency may also occur in patients with periprosthetic infection [117]. As a result, it increased mortality rates. Nowadays, the incidence of deep infection after TKA varies between 0.4 and 2% [74]. Factors that pave the way for infection in the postoperative period include the presence of rheumatoid arthritis, diabetes, hemophilia, malignancy, HIV, obesity, smoking, intravenous drug addiction, knee septic arthritis and osteomyelitis, prolonged surgical time, malnutrition, steroid use, and prolonged skin problems.

Antibiotic prophylaxis is the most effective method to prevent infection [118]. Prophylaxis should be administered 30–60 minutes. Before skin incision [119]. It has been shown that short postoperative antibiotherapy is more beneficial than the longer one [120].

Fewer people entering the operating room, using drapes to prevent superficial contamination, providing laminar air flow, effective sterilization of surgical instruments, and keeping the surgical time 150 minutes below are also necessary to prevent infection [121].

Risk groups of patients should be identified before the operation, and a separate planning should be made for each patient according to comorbid diseases. Antibiotic cement has been shown to reduce the infection rate in patients at risk [122]. However, it has been reported that the use of antibiotic cement in the patient group with no risk may cause premature loosening [123].

The most common organisms produced after infected knee arthroplasties are *Staphylococcus aureus*, coagulase negative *Staphylococcus*, and *Streptococcus* bacteria [124]. However, many microorganisms can also be active. Variations have occurred in microorganisms due to the unnecessary antibiotics used recently, and this has led to the development of resistance. Of these microorganisms, the most common isolates are methicillin-resistant *Staphylococcus aureus* (MRSA) and many antibiotics [125]. Fungal infections are not common, but the most common causative agents in these isolated are *Candida* species [126].

Bacteria that cause prosthetic infection form a biofilm layer on the implant. This biofilm layer increases the virulence of the agent. In addition, it forms resistance to treatment because of its limitation on antibiotic permeability. The best antibiotic to cross the biofilm layer is rifampicin [127]. There are studies suggesting the addition of rifampicin to antibiotic treatment specific for the reproductive bacteria [127, 128].

4.3.1 Diagnosis

Detailed anamnesis and detailed physical examination should be performed in the diagnosis of periprosthetic infection. In addition, the presence of a progressive radiolucent area around the prosthesis with direct radiographs, osteopenia, or osteolysis extending to the subchondral bone and the formation of new bone in the periosteal area can be evaluated in favor of infection [129]. The pain caused by rest is unique. However, increasing severity of pain and prolonged drainage at the wound site can also be evaluated in favor of infection. Arthrocentesis is then performed. In the case of active isolation, the necessary treatment is started. Empirical antibiotic therapy should be avoided. Wait until the agent is isolated.

Because empirical antibiotherapy will suppress a possible infection and may cause deep infection due to delayed diagnosis of prosthesis infection that may be saved by debridement and may require removal of the prosthesis [130].

CRP and sedimentation values should be evaluated in diagnosis. However, it should be remembered that CRP returns to its previous level after 14–21 days postoperatively [131]. Alpha defensin, lactoferrin, ELA-2, BPI, procalcitonin, and synovial CRP values are other parameters that can be used in diagnosis [132].

Current consensus has been reached in the diagnosis of periprosthetic infection [133]. Accordingly:

- Major criteria
  - Generation of the same agent in two positive cultures.
  - Presence of sinus mouth associated with prosthesis. In the presence of one of them, the diagnosis is established [133].
- Minor criteria
  - Calculated weights of high serum CRP (>1 mg/dL), D-dimer (>860 ng/mL), and erythrocyte sedimentation rate (>30 mm/h) are also 2, 2, and 1 points, respectively.
  - High synovial fluid white cell count (>3000 cells/μL), alpha defensin (signal cutoff ratio > 1), leukocyte esterase (++), polymorphonuclear percentage (>80%), and synovial CRP (>6.9 mg/L) were arranged as 3, 3, 3, 2, and 1 points, respectively.

Patients with a total score equal to or greater than 6 were considered infected.

4.3.2 Treatment

The goal of infection treatment in total knee arthroplasty is eradication of the infection, pain relief, and maintenance of limb function. Treatment options are antibiotic pressure, debridement, single- or double-stage revision, arthrodesis, resection arthroplasty, and amputation. Revision surgery also has single-stage or double-stage revision options [134–136].

4.4 Periprosthetic fractures

Periprosthetic fractures around the knee are fractures that occur during or after surgery within 15 cm of the knee joint or within 5 cm of the intramedullary part of the prosthesis, if any [137]. The incidence of these fractures after TKA is 0.3–2.5% for femur and 0.4 01% for tibia [138, 139].

The main risk factor related to the patient is the age of the patient. This risk is due to an increased risk of falling due to the patient's age and osteoporosis associated with age [140]. Corticosteroid use, diseases that may increase the risk of falling with rheumatoid arthritis (epilepsy, Parkinson's, cerebellar ataxia, myasthenia gravis) can be counted as other patient-related risk factors [141].

Intraoperative diaphyseal femoral fractures may occur due to incorrect placement of the intramedullary guide and osteopenia [142]. Unsuitable bone incisions, aggressive impaction of the ligamentous posterior stabilized femoral component, and eccentric placement of trial components are also risk factors for femoral fracture. It has been shown to increase the frequency of periprosthetic fractures due to increased resistance in flexion and rotation movements in anterior femoral notching [143]. The possibility of periprosthetic fracture is increased in revision TKA cases [144]. Periprosthetic fractures are more common due to the rotational forces of restrictive prosthesis using shear forces in the prosthesis [141].

Due to the stronger structure of the tibia, fracture development is rare.

For femoral periprosthetic fractures, there is a classification that questions fracture displacement and component fixation.

- Type 1 describes fractures with non-displaced and stable components.
- Type 2 refers to component stable fractures with displacement of more than 5 mm or angulation of more than 5°.
- Type 3 indicates loose fractures [145].

4.4.1 Treatment

4.4.1.1 Femoral fractures during surgery

The femur fractures vertically more than the metaphyseal region. A stable periosteum prevents displacement. It is followed conservatively without any additional intervention. For fractures penetrating the femoral cortex, whether or not a bone graft is used, the penetration level should be treated with a stem prosthesis that is at least twice the diameter of the femoral canal [146].

4.4.1.2 Postoperative femoral fractures

When non-displaced fractures and stable prosthesis occur after TKA, conservative treatment may be preferred. Four to six weeks of non-weight procedure, long leg plaster, or hinged orthosis is followed.

Displaced and unreducible supracondylar fractures are almost always treated surgically in the presence of adequate bone stock (**Figure 1**) [147].

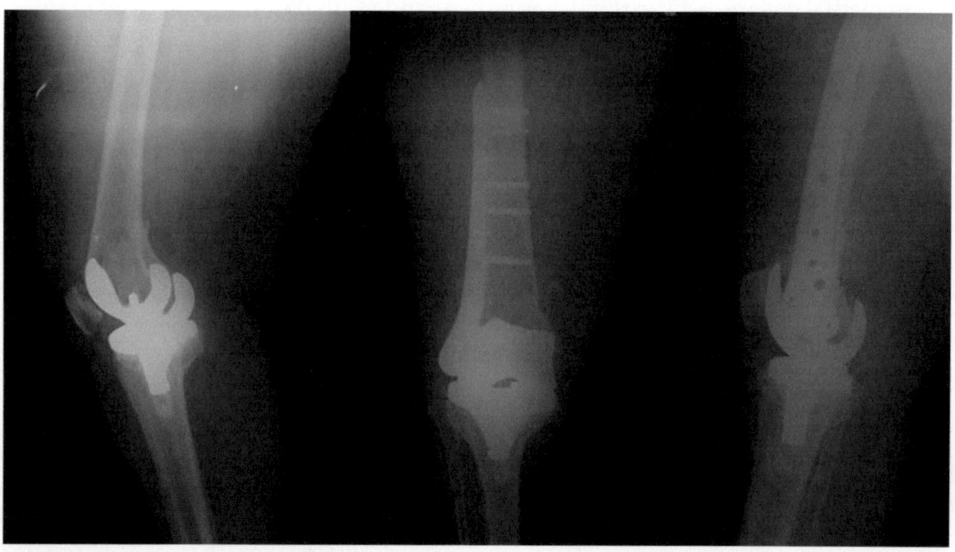

Figure 1.
Supracondylar periprosthetic femur fracture treated with open reduction and internal fixation.

Locked compression plates are preferred for knee periprosthetic fractures [144]. Prosthetic revision should be performed in fractures that cause prosthesis loosening and malposition. In these cases, stented prosthesis of sufficient length should be placed to obtain a stable fixation of the intact bone [138]. Knee replacement revision after periprosthetic fractures is often associated with the loss of range of motion (ROM) [148].

4.4.1.3 Tibia fractures

The majority of tibial periprosthetic fractures during surgery involve the plateau region and are generally non-displaced [146, 149]. If prosthetic loosening is present, revision surgery using a stem component long enough to cross the fracture line is required [150].

Postoperative tibial fractures can be examined in four groups. In type 1 fracture, revision is recommended because tibial component will be in varus alignment. The medial defect should be closed with bone graft or metal support [150]. Type 2 fractures are treated with nonsurgical treatment if the component is stable and there is minimal displacement [149]. Displaced type 2 fractures are treated with internal fixation. If the component is unstable, it must be revised using a long tibial stem to cross the fracture line [149]. Internal fixation should be performed for type 3 and 4 fractures [145].

4.5 Aseptic loosening

The deterioration of the relationship between prosthesis and bone is defined as loosening. The loosening may be between the prosthetic cement and the cement bone. Loosening is inevitable in long-term prostheses. It is useful to distinguish the concepts of osteolysis and loosening. Without prosthesis osteolysis, loosening of the cement may occur. The mechanisms that cause loosening are micromotion, component collapse, and periprosthetic osteolysis [151].

Overuse and osteopenia are the causes of patient-related loosening. Implant design may also be the cause of loosening. According to this, loosening is more likely in cementless prosthesis and constrained prosthesis. One of the most important causes of aseptic loosening is malalignment. It has been shown that a 4 mm medial collapse of the tibial component and varus deformity of more than 2° increases the likelihood of loosening [152]. In the early period, a radiolucent line is seen between the component and bone on radiography, and a collapse occurs as the loosening progresses. Loosening is more common around the tibial component [152]. In the presence of loosening around the whole component, septic loosening should be considered, and differential diagnosis should be performed.

In the case of loosening, the treatment is decided according to symptoms and progress. If pain is associated with instability and there are X-ray findings, early revision surgery is recommended for bone stock preservation.

4.6 Osteolysis

Osteolysis usually occurs due to inflammatory reactions caused by worn polyethylene particles or in the presence of infection. Metal particles can also cause osteolysis. Titanium causes more osteolysis than cobalt and chromium. Giant cells that develop against abrasive particles act by forming a membrane [153]. Particle size is important for this mechanism. The particle sizes range from 1 to 100 micrometers under the electron microscope. Large parts do not cause osteolysis [153]. There is no osteolysis if the parts are not spread to the cancellous bone, so osteolysis is not seen when the cancellous bone is properly covered with cement [154]. On the other hand, the incidence of osteolysis increases when pres-fit prosthesis is applied; screw fixation without cement is used or cement breaks [155]. Osteolysis is closely related to prosthetic design. Osteolysis usually occurs after 2 years of TKA. Occurrence is rare before 2 years [156]. Osteolysis is mostly seen in the tibia [157]. Diagnosis includes pain, joint effusion, and synovitis due to joint instability. Focal bone destruction may be seen on radiolucent line and X-ray. It can be seen that there is no continuity of trabeculae and bone cortex in cancellous bone. Therefore, control X-rays are very important in patient follow-up and must be compared with old radiographs in controls. CT and MRI can be used for osteolysis that cannot be detected on direct radiography [158].

If the lesion is small in treatment and the prosthesis is stable, observation is sufficient. Bisphosphonate and calcium supplementation can be initiated [159]. If the prosthesis is instable, two options can be applied. The first one is debridement, polyethylene replacement, and curettage, followed by impaction of the defect with bone graft. The second is revision [159].

4.7 Patellofemoral joint problems

Patellofemoral joint problems after TKA generally cause anterior knee pain. Patients' ability to tolerate this pain rarely causes patellofemoral joint problems to be revised [160]. It should be kept in mind that not only patellar component-related procedures but also procedures involving the tibiofemoral joint may cause this problem. Even in revision surgery due to a problem of patellofemoral origin, it is often caused by a component in the tibia and femur [161]. In a study, patella and malrotation were among the eight most common causes of failed TKA [162].

Advanced valgus alignment, previous high tibial osteotomy, or tuberositas tibia osteotomy increases the rate of patellofemoral joint problems in TKA [160].

There are many points to be considered in the surgical technique to prevent patellofemoral joint problems. These are [163]:

- *Component placement*: If the femoral component is placed medially, anteriorly, or flexed, or if there is internal rotation and if the component is excessive in size, patellofemoral problems may occur finally. Likewise, the medialization and internal rotation of the tibial component increases the risk.

- *Surgical approach type*: Midvastus and subvastus interventions that protect the extensor mechanism more can reduce PF joint problems.

- *Lateral release*: The need for lateral retinacular release increases PF joint problems.

- *Patella resection amount*: When patellar component is used, resection of the patella with anterior–posterior reduction of 12 mm increases the risk of PF joint problems [164, 165].

Patellar surface replacement is controversial today. However, in a recent study, it was found that anterior knee pain was less common in patients who underwent patellar surface change than those who did not. In the same study, the causes of PF joint revision were more common in patients without patella surface changes [166].

The results in patients with patellar articular surface alteration due to persistent anterior knee pain after TKA are not as successful as those with surface replacement during primary TKA [167]. In the treatment of anterior knee pain after TKA, mechanical causes should be investigated after the exclusion of an underlying infection.

Author details

Muhammet Salih AYAS[1], Muhammet Kalkışım[2*], Ahmet Köse[1] and Orkun Gül[2]

1 Orthopedics and Traumatology, University of Health Sciences, Erzurum Regional Training and Research Hospital, Turkey

2 Department of Orthopedics and Traumatology, Karadeniz Technical University, Turkey

*Address all correspondence to: muhammetkalkisim@gmail.com

References

[1] Healy WL, Della Valle CJ, Iorio R, Berend KR, Cushner FD, Dalury DF, et al. Complications of total knee arthroplasty: Standardized list and definitions of the knee society. Clinical Orthopaedics and Related Research. 2013;**471**:215-220. DOI: 10.1007/s11999-012-2489-y

[2] Dalury DF, Pomeroy DL, Gorab RS, Adams MJ. Why are total knee arthroplasties being revised? The Journal of Arthroplasty. 2013;**28**:120-121. DOI: 10.1016/j.arth.2013.04.051

[3] Langkamer V. Local vascular complications after knee replacement: A review with illustrative case reports. The Knee. 2001;**8**:259-264. DOI: 10.1016/S0968-0160(01)00103-X

[4] Abularrage CJ, Weiswasser JM, DeZee KJ, Slidell MB, Henderson WG, Sidawy AN. Predictors of lower extremity arterial injury after total knee or total hip arthroplasty. Journal of Vascular Surgery. 2008;**47**:803-807. DOI: 10.1016/J.JVS.2007.11.067

[5] Shoenfeld NA, Stuchin SA, Pearl R, Haveson S. The management of vascular injuries associated with total hip arthroplasty. Journal of Vascular Surgery. 1990;**11**:549-555. DOI: 10.1016/0741-5214(90)90301-P

[6] Calligaro KD, Dougherty MJ, Ryan S, Booth RE. Acute arterial complications associated with total hip and knee arthroplasty. Journal of Vascular Surgery. 2003;**38**:1170-1175. DOI: 10.1016/S0741-5214(03)00918-2

[7] Smith DE, McGraw RW, Taylor DC, Masri BA. Arterial complications and total knee arthroplasty. The Journal of the American Academy of Orthopaedic Surgeons. n.d.;**9**:253-257

[8] Rand JA. Vascular complications of total knee arthroplasty. Report of three cases. Journal of Arthroplasty. 1987;**2**:89-93

[9] Inomata K, Sekiya I, Otabe K, Nakamura T, Horie M, Koga H, et al. Acute arterial occlusion after total knee arthroplasty: A case report. Clinical Case Reports. 2017;**5**:1376-1380. DOI: 10.1002/ccr3.1075

[10] Saleh KJ, Hoeffel DP, Kassim RA, Burstein G. Complications after revision total knee arthroplasty. The Journal of Bone and Joint Surgery. American Volume. 2003;**85-A**(Suppl 1):S71-S74. DOI: 10.2106/00004623-200300001-00013

[11] Ninomiya JT, Dean JC, Goldberg VM. Injury to the popliteal artery and its anatomic location in total knee arthroplasty. The Journal of Arthroplasty. 1999;**14**:803-809

[12] Rubash HE, Berger RA, Britton CA, Nettrour WS, Seel MJ. Avoiding neurologic and vascular injuries with screw fixation of the tibial component in total knee arthroplasty. Clinical Orthopaedics and Related Research. 1993:56-63

[13] Rama KRBS. Timing of tourniquet release in knee arthroplasty: Meta-analysis of randomized, controlled trials. The Journal of Bone and Joint Surgery. 2007;**89**:699. DOI: 10.2106/JBJS.F.00497

[14] Holmberg A, Milbrink J, Berqqvist D. Arterial complications after knee arthroplasty: 4 cases and a review of the literature. Acta Orthopaedica Scandinavica. 01 Feb 1996;**67**(1):75-78. DOI: 10.3109/17453679608995616

[15] Ibrahim M, Booth RE, Clark TWI. Embolization of traumatic pseudoaneurysms after total knee arthroplasty. The Journal of Arthroplasty. 2004;**19**:123-128

[16] Kapetanos GA, Papavasiliou KA, Makris V, Nikolaides AP, Kirkos JM, Symeonides PP. Recurrent spontaneous hemarthrosis after total knee arthroplasty successfully treated with synoviorthesis. The Journal of Arthroplasty. 2008;**23**(6):931-933. DOI: 10.1016/j.arth.2007.07.012

[17] Knutson K, Leden I, Sturfelt G, Rosén I, Lidgren L. Nerve palsy after knee arthroplasty in patients with rheumatoid arthritis. Scandinavian Journal of Rheumatology. 1983;**12**:201-205

[18] Rose HA, Hood RW, Otis JC, Ranawat CS, Insall JN. Peroneal-nerve palsy following total knee arthroplasty. A review of the hospital for special surgery experience. The Journal of Bone and Joint Surgery. American Volume. 1982;**64**:347-351

[19] Horlocker TT, Hebl JR, Gali B, Jankowski CJ, Burkle CM, Berry DJ, et al. Anesthetic, patient, and surgical risk factors for neurologic complications after prolonged total tourniquet time during total knee arthroplasty. Anesthesia and Analgesia. 2006;**102**:950-955. DOI: 10.1213/01.ane.0000194875.05587.7e

[20] Black R, Green C, Sochart D. Postoperative numbness of the knee following total knee arthroplasty. Annals of the Royal College of Surgeons of England. 2013:565-568. DOI: 10.1308/003588413X13629960049009

[21] Idusuyi OB, Morrey BF. Peroneal nerve palsy after total knee arthroplasty. Assessment of predisposing and prognostic factors. The Journal of Bone and Joint Surgery. American Volume. 1996;**78**:177-184. DOI: 10.2106/00004623-199602000-00003.

[22] Brull R, McCartney CJL, Chan VWS, El-Beheiry H. Neurological complications after regional anesthesia: Contemporary estimates of risk. Anesthesia and Analgesia. 2007;**104**:965-974. DOI: 10.1213/01.ane.0000258740.17193.ec

[23] Hopton BP, Tommichan MC, Howell FR. Reducing lateral skin flap numbness after total knee arthroplasty. The Knee. 2004;**11**:289-291. DOI: 10.1016/j.knee.2003.09.004

[24] Nam D, Abdel MP, Cross MB, LaMont LE, Reinhardt KR, McArthur BA, et al. The management of extensor mechanism complications in total knee arthroplasty: AAOS exhibit selection. The Journal of Bone and Joint Surgery. 2014;**96**(6):e47. DOI: 10.2106/JBJS.M.00949

[25] Parker DA, Dunbar MJ, Rorabeck CH. Extensor mechanism failure associated with total knee arthroplasty: Prevention and management. The Journal of the American Academy of Orthopaedic Surgeons. 2003;**11**:238-247

[26] Rand J, Morrey B, Bryan R. Patellar tendon rupture after total knee arthroplasty. Clinical Orthopaedics and Related Research. 1989;**246**:233-238

[27] Schoderbek RJ, Brown TE, Mulhall KJ, Mounasamy V, Iorio R, Krackow KA, et al. Extensor mechanism disruption after total knee arthroplasty. Clinical Orthopaedics and Related Research. 2006;**446**:176-185. DOI: 10.1097/01.blo.0000218726.06473.26

[28] Putman S, Boureau F, Girard J, Migaud H, Pasquier G. Patellar complications after total knee arthroplasty. Orthopaedics and Traumatology, Surgery and Research. 2019;**105**:S43-S51. DOI: 10.1016/j.otsr.2018.04.028

[29] Browne JA, Hanssen AD. Reconstruction of patellar tendon disruption after total knee arthroplasty: Results of a new technique utilizing synthetic mesh. The Journal of Bone

and Joint Surgery. American Volume. 2011;**93**:1137-1143. DOI: 10.2106/JBJS.J.01036

[30] Ayas MS, Gül O, Okutan AE, Turhan AU. Extensor mechanism reconstruction with peroneus longus tendon autograft for neglected patellar fracture, report of 2 cases. Journal of Clinical Orthopaedics and Trauma. 2019;**10**:S226-S230. DOI: 10.1016/j.jcot.2019.05.020

[31] Dobbs RE, Hanssen AD, Lewallen DG, Pagnano MW. Quadriceps tendon rupture after total knee arthroplasty: Prevalence, complications, and outcomes. The Journal of Bone and Joint Surgery. 2005;**87**(1):37-45. DOI: 10.2106/JBJS.D.01910

[32] Hozack WJ, Goll SR, Lotke PA, Rothman RH, Booth RE. The treatment of patellar fractures after total knee arthroplasty. Clinical Orthopaedics and Related Research. 1988;**236**:123-127

[33] Ortiguera CJ, Berry DJ. Patellar fracture after total knee arthroplasty. Journal of Bone and Joint Surgery. 2002;**84**(4):532-540

[34] Chalidis BE, Tsiridis E, Tragas AA, Stavrou Z, Giannoudis PV. Management of periprosthetic patellar fractures. A systematic review of literature. Injury. 2007. DOI: 10.1016/j.injury.2007.02.054

[35] Leopold MSS, McStay C, Klafeta K, Jacobs JJ, Berger RA, Rosenberg AG. Primary repair of intraoperative disruption of the medial collateral ligament during total knee arthroplasty. The Journal of Bone and Joint Surgery. 2001. DOI: 10.2106/00004623-200101000-00012

[36] Healy WL, Della Valle CJ, Iorio R, Berend KR, Cushner FD, Dalury DF, et al. Complications of total knee arthroplasty: Standardized list and definitions of the knee society knee. Clinical Orthopaedics and Related Research. 2013. DOI: 10.1007/s11999-012-2489-y

[37] Lee GC, Lotke PA. Management of intraoperative medial collateral ligament injury during TKA. Clinical Orthopaedics and Related Research. 2011. DOI: 10.1007/s11999-010-1502-6

[38] Wang X, Liu H, Cao P, Liu C, Dong Z, Qi J, et al. Clinical outcomes of medial collateral ligament injury in total knee arthroplasty. Medicine (United States). 2017. DOI: 10.1097/MD.0000000000007617

[39] Kenneth Della Torre P, Stephens A, Lii H. Management of medial collateral ligament injury during primary total knee arthroplasty: A systematic review. Reconstructive Review. 2014;**4**:17-23. DOI: 10.15438/rr.v4i2.69

[40] Adravanti P, Dini F, Calafiore G, Rosa MA. Medial collateral ligament reconstruction during TKA: A new approach and surgical technique. Joints. 2015;**3**(04):215-217. DOI: 10.11138/jts/2015.3.4.215

[41] Whiteside LA. Correction of ligament and bone defects in total arthroplasty of the severely valgus knee. Clinical Orthopaedics and Related Research. 1993;**288**:234-245

[42] Dimitris K, Taylor BC, Steensen RN. Excursion of oscillating saw blades in total knee arthroplasty. The Journal of Arthroplasty. 2010;**25**(1):158-160. DOI: 10.1016/j.arth.2008.09.021

[43] Zheng X, Li T, Wang J, Dong J, Gao S.Medial collateral ligament reconstruction using bone-patellar tendon-bone allograft for chronic medial knee instability combined with multi-ligament injuries: A new technique. Journal of Orthopaedic Surgery and Research. 2016;**11**:85. DOI: 10.1186/s13018-016-0416-8

[44] Heller K-D. Intraoperative damage to the medial collateral ligament (MCL)—what is to be done? Zeitschrift für Orthopädie und Unfallchirurgie. 2013;**151**:580-584. DOI: 10.1055/s-0033-1350932.

[45] Koo MH, Choi CH. Conservative treatment for the intraoperative detachment of medial collateral ligament from the tibial attachment site during primary total knee arthroplasty. The Journal of Arthroplasty. 2009;**24**(8):1249-1253. DOI: 10.1016/j.arth.2009.06.007

[46] Siqueira MBP, Haller K, Mulder A, Goldblum AS, Klika AK, Barsoum WK. Outcomes of medial collateral ligament injuries during total knee arthroplasty. The Journal of Knee Surgery. 2016;**29**:68-73. DOI: 10.1055/s-0034-1394166

[47] Kotzé A, Carter LA, Scally AJ. Effect of a patient blood management programme on preoperative anaemia, transfusion rate, and outcome after primary hip or knee arthroplasty: A quality improvement cycle. British Journal of Anaesthesia. 2012;**108**(6):943-952. DOI: 10.1093/bja/aes135

[48] Raut VV, Stone MH, Wroblewski BM. Reduction of postoperative blood loss after press-fit condylar knee arthroplasty with use of a femoral intramedullary plug. The Journal of Bone and Joint Surgery. American Volume. 1993;**75**:1356-1357. DOI: 10.2106/00004623-199309000-00010

[49] Juelsgaard P, Larsen UT, Sørensen JV, Madsen F, Søballe K. Hypotensive epidural anesthesia in total knee replacement without tourniquet: Reduced blood loss and transfusion. Regional Anesthesia and Pain Medicine. n.d.;**26**:105-110. DOI: 10.1053/rapm.2001.21094

[50] Gibbons CE, Solan MC, Ricketts DM, Patterson M. Cryotherapy compared with Robert Jones bandage after total knee replacement: A prospective randomized trial. International Orthopaedics. 2001;**25**:250-252. DOI: 10.1007/s002640100227

[51] Wang GJ, Hungerford DS, Savory CG, Rosenberg AG, Mont MA, Burks SG, et al. Use of fibrin sealant to reduce bloody drainage and hemoglobin loss after total knee arthroplasty: A brief note on a randomized prospective trial. The Journal of Bone and Joint Surgery. American Volume. 2001;**83**:1503-1505. DOI: 10.2106/00004623-200110000-00007

[52] Prasad N, Padmanabhan V, Mullaji A. Comparison between two methods of drain clamping after total knee arthroplasty. Archives of Orthopaedic and Trauma Surgery. 2005;**125**:381-384. DOI: 10.1007/s00402-005-0813-7

[53] Roy N, Smith M, Anwar M, Elsworth C. Delayed release of drain in total knee replacement reduces blood loss. A prospective randomised study. Acta Orthopaedica Belgica. 2006;**72**:34-38

[54] Ryu J, Sakamoto A, Honda T, Saito S. The postoperative drain-clamping method for hemostasis in total knee arthroplasty. Reducing postoperative bleeding in total knee arthroplasty. Bulletin/Hospital for Joint Diseases. 1997;**56**:251-254

[55] Charoencholvanich K, Siriwattanasakul P. Tranexamic acid reduces blood loss and blood transfusion after TKA: A prospective randomized controlled trial. Clinical Orthopaedics and Related Research. 2011;**469**:2874-2880. DOI: 10.1007/s11999-011-1874-2

[56] Janssens M, Joris J, David JL, Lemaire R, Lamy M. High-dose

aprotinin reduces blood loss in patients undergoing total hip replacement surgery. Anesthesiology. 1994;**80**:23-29. DOI: 10.1097/00000542-199401000-00007

[57] Dubber AH, McNicol GP, Douglas AS. Amino-methyl-cyclohexane-carboxylicacid: AMCHA; a new patent inhibitor of the fibrinolysis. British Journal of Haematology. 1965

[58] Sano M, Hakusui H, Kojima C, Akimoto T. Absorption and excretion of tranexamic acid following intravenous, intramuscular and oral administrations in healthy volunteers. Rinsho Yakuri/Japanese Journal of Clinical Pharmacology and Therapeutics. 1976. DOI: 10.3999/jscpt.7.375

[59] Molloy DO, Archbold HAP, Ogonda L, McConway J, Wilson RK, Beverland DE. Comparison of topical fibrin spray and tranexamic acid on blood loss after total knee replacement. Journal of Bone and Joint Surgery. British Volume (London). 2007. DOI: 10.1302/0301-620x.89b3.17565

[60] Veien M, Sørensen JV, Madsen F, Juelsgaard P. Tranexamic acid given intraoperatively reduces blood loss after total knee replacement: A randomized, controlled study. Acta Anaesthesiologica Scandinavica. 2002;**46**:1206-1211

[61] Orpen NM, Little C, Walker G, Crawfurd EJP. Tranexamic acid reduces early post-operative blood loss after total knee arthroplasty: A prospective randomised controlled trial of 29 patients. The Knee. 2006;**13**:106-110. DOI: 10.1016/j.knee.2005.11.001

[62] Jansen AJ, Andreica S, Claeys M, D'Haese J, Camu F, Jochmans K. Use of tranexamic acid for an effective blood conservation strategy after total knee arthroplasty. British Journal of Anaesthesia. 1999;**83**(4):596-601. DOI: 10.1093/bja/83.4.596

[63] Feng B, Lin J, Jin J, Qian W-W, Wang W, Weng X-S. Thirty-day postoperative complications following primary total knee arthroplasty: A retrospective study of incidence and risk factors at a single Center in China. Chinese Medical Journal. 2017;**130**:2551-2556. DOI: 10.4103/0366-6999.213071

[64] Parvizi J, Mui A, Purtill JJ, Sharkey PF, Hozack WJ, Rothman RH. Total joint arthroplasty: When do fatal or near-fatal complications occur? The Journal of Bone and Joint Surgery. American Volume. 2007;**89**:27-32. DOI: 10.2106/JBJS.E.01443

[65] Simons MJ, Amin NH, Scuderi GR. Acute wound complications after total knee arthroplasty: Prevention and management. The Journal of the American Academy of Orthopaedic Surgeons. 2017;**25**:547-555. DOI: 10.5435/JAAOS-D-15-00402

[66] Galat DD, McGovern SC, Larson DR, Harrington JR, Hanssen AD, Clarke HD. Surgical treatment of early wound complications following primary total knee arthroplasty. The Journal of Bone and Joint Surgery. 2009;**91**(1):48-54. DOI: 10.2106/JBJS.G.01371

[67] Stryker LS, Abdel MP, Morrey ME, Morrow MM, Kor DJ, Morrey BF. Elevated postoperative blood glucose and preoperative hemoglobin A1C are associated with increased wound complications following total joint arthroplasty. The Journal of Bone and Joint Surgery. American Volume. 2013;**95**:808-814, S1-2. DOI: 10.2106/JBJS.L.00494

[68] Simons MJ, Nirav HA, Giles RS. Acute wound complications after total knee arthroplasty: Prevention and management. Journal of the American Academy of Orthopaedic Surgeons; 2017;**25**(8):547-555

[69] Osei DA, Rebehn KA, Boyer MI. Soft-tissue defects after

total knee arthroplasty: Management and reconstruction. The Journal of the American Academy of Orthopaedic Surgeons. 2016;**24**:769-779. DOI: 10.5435/JAAOS-D-15-00241

[70] Ries MD. Skin necrosis after total knee arthroplasty. The Journal of Arthroplasty. 2002;**17**(4):74-77. DOI: 10.1054/arth.2002.32452

[71] Vince KG, Abdeen A. Total knee replacement after valgus tibial osteotomy. Technical problems. Clinical Orthopaedics and Related Research. 1992;**78**(7):438-448

[72] Gaine WJ, Ramamohan NA, Hussein NA, Hullin MG, McCreath SW. Wound infection in hip and knee arthroplasty. Journal of Bone and Joint Surgery. British Volume (London). 2000;**82**:561-565

[73] Wu C-T, Chen I-L, Wang J-W, Ko J-Y, Wang C-J, Lee C-H. Surgical site infection after total knee arthroplasty: Risk factors in patients with timely administration of systemic prophylactic antibiotics. The Journal of Arthroplasty. 2016;**31**:1568-1573. DOI: 10.1016/j.arth.2016.01.017

[74] Blom AW, Brown J, Taylor AH, Pattison G, Whitehouse S, Bannister GC. Infection after total knee arthroplasty. Journal of Bone and Joint Surgery. British Volume (London). 2004;**86**(5):688-691

[75] Namba RS, Paxton L, Fithian DC, Lou SM. Obesity and perioperative morbidity in total hip and total knee arthroplasty patients. The Journal of Arthroplasty. 2005;**20**:46-50. DOI: 10.1016/j.arth.2005.04.023

[76] Bongartz T, Halligan CS, Osmon DR, Reinalda MS, Bamlet WR, Crowson CS, et al. Incidence and risk factors of prosthetic joint infection after total hip or knee replacement in patients with rheumatoid arthritis. Arthritis Care and Research. 2008;**59**(12):1713-1720. DOI: 10.1002/art.24060

[77] Papavasiliou AV, Isaac DL, Marimuthu R, Skyrme A, Armitage A. Infection in knee replacements after previous injection of intra-articular steroid. Journal of Bone and Joint Surgery. British Volume (London). 2006;**88**:321-323. DOI: 10.1302/0301-620X.88B3.17136.

[78] Hijas-Gómez AI, Lucas WC, Checa-García A, Martínez-Martín J, Fahandezh-Saddi H, Gil-de-Miguel Á, et al. Surgical site infection incidence and risk factors in knee arthroplasty: A 9-year prospective cohort study at a university teaching hospital in Spain. American Journal of Infection Control. 2018;**46**:1335-1340. DOI: 10.1016/j.ajic.2018.06.010

[79] Saleh K, Olson M, Resig S, Bershadsky B, Kuskowski M, Gioe T, et al. Predictors of wound infection in hip and knee joint replacement: Results from a 20 year surveillance program. Journal of Orthopaedic Research. 2002;**20**:506-515. DOI: 10.1016/S0736-0266(01)00153-X

[80] Teo BJX, Yeo W, Chong HC, Tan AHC. Surgical site infection after primary total knee arthroplasty is associated with a longer duration of surgery. Journal of Orthopaedic Surgery. 2018:**26**(2). DOI: 10.1177/2309499018785647

[81] Scuderi GR. Avoiding postoperative wound complications in total joint arthroplasty. The Journal of Arthroplasty. 2018;**33**:3109-3112. DOI: 10.1016/j.arth.2018.01.025

[82] Löwik CAM, Wagenaar F-C, van der Weegen W, Poolman RW, Nelissen RGHH, Bulstra SK, et al. LEAK study: Design of a nationwide randomised controlled trial to find the best way to treat wound leakage after primary hip and knee arthroplasty. BMJ

Open. 2017;7:e018673. DOI: 10.1136/bmjopen-2017-018673

[83] Haleem AA, Berry DJ, Hanssen AD. Mid-term to long-term followup of two-stage reimplantation for infected total knee arthroplasty. Clinical Orthopaedics and Related Research. 2004;**428**:35-39. DOI: 10.1097/01.blo.0000147713.64235.73

[84] Özkurt B, Utkan A. Primer total diz artroplastisi sonrası yara yeri sorunları ve yüzeyel enfeksiyon. TOTBID Dergisi. 2019;**18**:128-137. DOI: 10.14292/totbid.dergisi.2019.15

[85] Segal JB, Eng J, Tamariz LJ, Bass EB. Review of the evidence on diagnosis of deep venous thrombosis and pulmonary embolism. Annals of Family Medicine. 2003;**5**:63-73. DOI: 10.1370/afm.648

[86] Shahi A, Chen AF, Tan TL, Maltenfort MG, Kucukdurmaz F, Parvizi J. The incidence and economic burden of in-hospital venous thromboembolism in the United States. The Journal of Arthroplasty. 2017;**32**:1063-1066. DOI: 10.1016/j.arth.2016.10.020

[87] Dorr LD, Gendelman V, Maheshwari AV, Boutary M, Wan Z, Long WT. Multimodal thrombo prophylaxis for total hip and knee arthroplasty based on risk assessment. The Journal of Bone and Joint Surgery. American Volume. 2007;**89**:2648-2657. DOI: 10.2106/JBJS.F.00235

[88] Ogonda L, Hill J, Doran E, Dennison J, Stevenson M, Beverland D. Aspirin for thromboprophylaxis after primary lower limb arthroplasty: Early thromboembolic events and 90 day mortality in 11,459 patients. The Bone and Joint Journal. 2016;**98-B**:341-348. DOI: 10.1302/0301-620X.98B3.36511

[89] Tun NM, Oo TH. Prevention and treatment of venous thromboembolism with new oral anticoagulants: A practical update for clinicians. Thrombosis. 2013;**2013**:10. Article ID: 183616. DOI: 10.1155/2013/183616

[90] Anderson FA, Wheeler HB, Goldberg RJ, Hosmer DW, Patwardhan NA, Jovanovic B, et al. A population-based perspective of the hospital incidence and case-fatality rates of deep vein thrombosis and pulmonary embolism. The Worcester DVT Study. Archives of Internal Medicine. 1991;**151**:933-938

[91] Fukuda A, Hasegawa M, Kato K, Shi D, Sudo A, Uchida A. Effect of tourniquet application on deep vein thrombosis after total knee arthroplasty. Archives of Orthopaedic and Trauma Surgery. 2007;**127**:671-675. DOI: 10.1007/s00402-006-0244-0

[92] Aglietti P, Baldini A, Vena LM, Abbate R, Fedi S, Falciani M. Effect of tourniquet use on activation of coagulation in total knee replacement. Clinical Orthopaedics and Related Research. 2000;**371**:169-177. DOI: 10.1097/00003086-200002000-00021

[93] Lieberman JR, Huo MM, Hanway J, Salvati EA, Sculco TP, Sharrock NE. The prevalence of deep venous thrombosis after total hip arthroplasty with hypotensive epidural anesthesia. The Journal of Bone and Joint Surgery. American Volume. 1994;**76**:341-348. DOI: 10.2106/00004623-199403000-00004

[94] Ho WK, Hankey GJ, Lee CH, Eikelboom JW. Venous thromboembolism: Diagnosis and management of deep venous thrombosis. The Medical Journal of Australia. 2005;**182**:476-481

[95] Geerts W, Heit J, Clagett G, Pineio G, Colwell C, Anderson F, et al. Prevention of venous thromboembolism: 6th ACCP consensus conference on antithrombotic

therapy. Chest Journal. 2001. DOI: 10.1378/chest.126.3_suppl.338S

[96] Goodacre S, Sampson F, Thomas S, van Beek E, Sutton A. Systematic review and meta-analysis of the diagnostic accuracy of ultrasonography for deep vein thrombosis. BMC Medical Imaging. 2005. DOI: 10.1186/1471-2342-5-6

[97] Wells PS, Anderson DR, Rodger M, Stiell I, Dreyer JF, Barnes D, et al. Excluding pulmonary embolism at the bedside without diagnostic imaging: Management of patients with suspected pulmonary embolism presenting to the emergency department by using a simple clinical model and d-dimer. Annals of Internal Medicine. 2001

[98] Pierce TP, Cherian JJ, Jauregui JJ, Elmallah RK, Lieberman JR, Mont MA. A current review of mechanical compression and its role in venous thromboembolic prophylaxis in total knee and total hip arthroplasty. The Journal of Arthroplasty. 2015;**30**:2279-2284. DOI: 10.1016/j.arth.2015.05.045

[99] Cafri G, Paxton EW, Chen Y, Cheetham CT, Gould MK, Sluggett J, et al. Comparative effectiveness and safety of drug prophylaxis for prevention of venous thromboembolism after total knee arthroplasty. The Journal of Arthroplasty. 2017;**32**:3524-3528.e1. DOI: 10.1016/j.arth.2017.05.042

[100] Bala A, Huddleston JI, Goodman SB, Maloney WJ, Amanatullah DF. Venous thromboembolism prophylaxis after TKA: Aspirin, warfarin, enoxaparin, or factor Xa inhibitors? Clinical Orthopaedics and Related Research. 2017;**475**:2205-2213. DOI: 10.1007/s11999-017-5394-6

[101] Gutowski CJ, Zmistowski BM, Lonner JH, Purtill JJ, Parvizi J. Direct costs of aspirin versus warfarin for venous thromboembolism prophylaxis after total knee or hip arthroplasty. The Journal of Arthroplasty. 2015;**30**:36-38. DOI: 10.1016/j.arth.2015.04.048

[102] Dalury DF, Pomeroy DL, Gorab RS, Adams MJ. Why are total knee arthroplasties being revised? The Journal of Arthroplasty. 2013;**28**:120-121. DOI: 10.1016/j.arth.2013.04.051

[103] Song SJ, Detch RC, Maloney WJ, Goodman SB, Huddleston JI. Causes of instability after total knee arthroplasty. The Journal of Arthroplasty. 2014;**29**:360-364. DOI: 10.1016/j.arth.2013.06.023

[104] Vince K. Mid-flexion instability after total knee arthroplasty woolly thinking or a real concern? The Bone and Joint Journal. 2016;**98(**1 SuppleA):84-88

[105] Matsuda S, Ito H. Ligament balancing in total knee arthroplasty - medial stabilizing technique. The Asia-Pacific Journal of Sports Medicine, Arthroscopy, Rehabilitation and Technology. 2015;**2**(4):108-113. DOI: 10.1016/j.asmart.2015.07.002

[106] Romero J, Stähelin T, Binkert C, Pfirrmann C, Hodler J, Kessler O. The clinical consequences of flexion gap asymmetry in total knee arthroplasty. The Journal of Arthroplasty. 2007;**22**:235-240. DOI: 10.1016/j.arth.2006.04.024

[107] Schiavone Panni A, Cerciello S, Vasso M, Tartarone M. Stiffness in total knee arthroplasty. Journal of Orthopaedics and Traumatology. 2009;**10**(3):111-118. DOI: 10.1007/s10195-009-0054-6

[108] Nelson CL, Kim J, Lotke PA. Stiffness after total knee arthroplasty. JBJS Essential Surgical Techniques. 2005;**os-87**:264-270. DOI: 10.2106/JBJS.E-00345

[109] Ritter MA, Harty LD, Davis KE, Meding JB, Berend ME. Predicting range

of motion after total knee arthroplasty. Clustering, log-linear regression, and regression tree analysis. The Journal of Bone and Joint Surgery. American Volume. 2003;**85**:1278-1285. DOI: 10.2106/00004623-200307000-00014

[110] Meehan JP, Monazzam S, Miles T, Danielsen B, White RH. Postoperative stiffness requiring manipulation under anesthesia is significantly reduced after simultaneous versus staged bilateral total knee arthroplasty. The Journal of Bone and Joint Surgery. American Volume. 2017;**99**:2085-2093. DOI: 10.2106/JBJS.17.00130

[111] Schurman DJ, Parker JN, Ornstein D. Total condylar knee replacement. A study of factors influencing range of motion as late as two years after arthroplasty. The Journal of Bone and Joint Surgery. American Volume. 1985;**67**:1006-1014

[112] Esler CNN, Lock K, Harper WMM, Gregg PJJ. Manipulation of total knee replacements. Is the flexion gained retained? The Journal of Bone and Joint Surgery. British volume. 1999;**81**(1):27-29. DOI: 10.1302/0301-620X.81B1.8848

[113] O'Driscoll SW, Giori NJ. Continuous passive motion (CPM): Theory and principles of clinical application. Journal of Rehabilitation Research and Development. 2000;**37**(2):179-188

[114] Scranton PE. Management of knee pain and stiffness after total knee arthroplasty. The Journal of Arthroplasty. 2001;**16**:428-435. DOI: 10.1054/arth.2001.22250

[115] Fitzsimmons SE, Vazquez EA, Bronson MJ. How to treat the stiff total knee arthroplasty? A systematic review. Clinical Orthopaedics and Related Research. 2010;**468**(4):1096-1106. DOI: 10.1007/s11999-010-1230-y

[116] Mont MA, Seyler TM, Marulanda GA, Delanois RE, Bhave A. Surgical treatment and customized rehabilitation for stiff knee arthroplasties. Clinical Orthopaedics and Related Research. 2006;**446**:193-200. DOI: 10.1097/01.blo.0000214419.36959.8c

[117] Hebert CK, Williams RE, Levy RS, Barrack RL. Cost of treating an infected total knee replacement. Clinical Orthopaedics and Related Research. 1996:140-145. DOI: 10.1097/00003086-199610000-00019

[118] Hill C, Flamant R, Mazas F, Evrard J. Prophylactic cefazolin versus placebo in total hip replacement. Report of a multicentre double-blind randomised trial. Lancet (London, England). 1981;**1**:795-796. DOI: 10.1016/s0140-6736(81)92678-7

[119] Leigh DA, Griggs J, Tighe CM, Powell HD, Church JC, Wise K, et al. Pharmacokinetic study of ceftazidime in bone and serum of patients undergoing hip and knee arthroplasty. The Journal of Antimicrobial Chemotherapy. 1985;**16**:637-642. DOI: 10.1093/jac/16.5.637

[120] Mauerhan DR, Nelson CL, Smith DL, Fitzgerald RH, Slama TG, Petty RW, et al. Prophylaxis against infection in total joint arthroplasty. One day of cefuroxime compared with three days of cefazolin. The Journal of Bone and Joint Surgery. American Volume. 1994;**76**:39-45. DOI: 10.2106/00004623-199401000-00006

[121] Peersman G, Laskin R, Davis J, Peterson M. Infection in total knee replacement: A retrospective review of 6489 total knee replacements. Clinical Orthopaedics and Related Research. 2001:15-23

[122] Jämsen E, Huhtala H, Puolakka T, Moilanen T. Risk factors for infection after knee arthroplasty. A register-based analysis of 43,149 cases. The Journal of

Bone and Joint Surgery. American Volume. 2009;**91**:38-47. DOI: 10.2106/JBJS.G.01686

[123] Hanssen AD. Prophylactic use of antibiotic bone cement: An emerging standard--in opposition. Journal of Arthroplasty. 2004;**19**:73-77

[124] Wasielewski RC, Barden RM, Rosenberg AG. Results of different surgical procedures on total knee arthroplasty infections. The Journal of Arthroplasty. 1996;**11**:931-938

[125] Kilgus DJ, Howe DJ, Strang A. Results of periprosthetic hip and knee infections caused by resistant bacteria. Clinical Orthopaedics and Related Research. 2002;**404**:116-124. DOI: 10.1097/00003086-200211000-00021

[126] Phelan DM, Osmon DR, Keating MR, Hanssen AD. Delayed reimplantation arthroplasty for candidal prosthetic joint infection: A report of 4 cases and review of the literature. Clinical Infectious Diseases. 2002;**34**:930-938. DOI: 10.1086/339212

[127] Zimmerli W, Widmer AF, Blatter M, Frei R, Ochsner PE. Role of rifampin for treatment of orthopedic implant-related staphylococcal infections: A randomized controlled trial. Foreign-body infection (FBI) study group. JAMA. 1998;**279**(19):1537-1541

[128] Arizono T, Oga M, Sugioka Y. Increased resistance of bacteria after adherence to polymethyl methacrylate. An in vitro study. Acta Orthopaedica Scandinavica. 1992;**63**:661-664

[129] Morrey BF, Westholm F, Schoifet S, Rand JA, Bryan RS. Long-term results of various treatment options for infected total knee arthroplasty. Clinical Orthopaedics and Related Research. 1989:120-128

[130] Schoifet SD, Morrey BF. Persistent infection after successful arthrodesis for infected total knee arthroplasty: A report of two cases. Journal of Arthroplasty. 1990;**5**(3):277-279. DOI: 10.1016/S0883-5403(08)80083-6

[131] White J, Kelly M, Dunsmuir R. C-reactive protein level after total hip and total knee replacement. Journal of Bone and Joint Surgery. British Volume (London). 1998;**80**:909-911

[132] Tahta M, Simsek ME, Isik C, Akkaya M, Gursoy S, Bozkurt M. Does inflammatory joint diseases affect the accuracy of infection biomarkers in patients with periprosthetic joint infections? A prospective comparative reliability study. Journal of Orthopaedic Science. 2019;**24**:286-289. DOI: 10.1016/j.jos.2018.08.022

[133] Parvizi J, Tan TL, Goswami K, Higuera C, Della Valle C, Chen AF, et al. The 2018 definition of Periprosthetic hip and knee infection: An evidence-based and validated criteria. The Journal of Arthroplasty. 2018;**33**:1309-1314.e2. DOI: 10.1016/j.arth.2018.02.078

[134] Shaikh AA, Ha CW, Park YG, Park YB. Two-stage approach to primary TKA in infected arthritic knees using intraoperatively molded articulating cement spacers. Clinical Orthopaedics and Related Research. 2014. DOI: 10.1007/s11999-014-3545-6

[135] Juul R, Fabrin J, Poulsen K, Schroder HM. Use of a new knee prosthesis as an articulating spacer in two-stage revision of infected total knee arthroplasty. The Knee Surgery and Related Research. 2016. DOI: 10.5792/ksrr.2016.28.3.239

[136] Ha C-W. Treatment of infected total knee arthroplasty. The Knee Surgery and Related Research. 2017. DOI: 10.5792/ksrr.17.301

[137] Dennis DA. Periprosthetic fractures following total knee arthroplasty. Instructional Course Lectures. 2001;**50**:379-389

[138] Ricci WM. Periprosthetic femur fractures. Journal of Orthopaedic Trauma. 2015. DOI: 10.1097/BOT.0000000000000282

[139] Haller JM, Kubiak EN, Spiguel A, Gardner MJ, Horwitz DS. Intramedullary nailing of tibial shaft fractures distal to total knee arthroplasty. Journal of Orthopaedic Trauma. 2014. DOI: 10.1097/BOT.0000000000000096

[140] Canton G, Ratti C, Fattori R, Hoxhaj B, Murena L. Periprosthetic knee fractures. A review of epidemiology, risk factors, diagnosis, management and outcome. Acta Biomedica. 2017. DOI: 10.23750/abm.v88i2 -S.6522

[141] Culp RW, Schmidt RG, Hanks G, Mak A, Esterhai JL, Heppenstall RB. Supracondylar fracture of the femur following prosthetic knee arthroplasty. Clinical Orthopaedics and Related Research. 1987;**222**:212-222

[142] Lombardi AV, Mallory TH, Waterman RA, Eberle RW. Intercondylar distal femoral fracture. An unreported complication of posterior-stabilized total knee arthroplasty. The Journal of Arthroplasty. 1995;**10**:643-650

[143] Gujarathi N, Putti AB, Abboud RJ, MacLean JGB, Espley AJ, Kellett CF. Risk of periprosthetic fracture after anterior femoral notching: A 9-year follow-up of 200 total knee arthroplasties. Acta Orthopaedica. 2009;**80**(5):553-556. DOI: 10.3109/17453670903350099

[144] Parvizi J, Jain N, Schmidt AH. Periprosthetic knee fractures. Journal of Orthopaedic Trauma. 2008;**22**:663-671. DOI: 10.1097/BOT.0b013e31816ed989

[145] Rorabeck CH, Taylor JW. Periprosthetic fractures of the femur complicating total knee arthroplasty. The Orthopedic Clinics of North America. 1999;**30**:265-277

[146] Engh GA, Ammeen DJ. Periprosthetic fractures adjacent to total knee implants: Treatment and clinical results. Instructional Course Lectures. 1998;**47**:437-448

[147] Merkel KD, Johnson EW. Supracondylar fracture of the femur after total knee arthroplasty. The Journal of Bone and Joint Surgery. American Volume. 1986;**68**:29-43

[148] Mortazavi SMJ, Kurd MF, Bender B, Post Z, Parvizi J, Purtill JJ. Distal femoral arthroplasty for the treatment of periprosthetic fractures after total knee arthroplasty. The Journal of Arthroplasty. 2010;**25**:775-780. DOI: 10.1016/j.arth.2009.05.024

[149] Felix NA, Stuart MJ, Hanssen AD. Periprosthetic fractures of the tibia associated with total knee arthroplasty. Clinical Orthopaedics and Related Research. 1997;**345**:113-124

[150] Rand JA, Coventry MB. Stress fractures after total knee arthroplasty. The Journal of Bone and Joint Surgery. American Volume. 1980;**62**:226-233

[151] Işık C, Emre F, Ertaş SE. Aseptik gevşeme. TOTBİD Dergisi. 2019;**18**:163-169. DOI: 10.14292/totbid.dergisi.2019.19

[152] Lee B-S, Cho H-I, Bin S-I, Kim J-M, Jo B-K. Femoral component varus malposition is associated with tibial aseptic loosening after TKA. Clinical Orthopaedics and Related Research. 2018;**476**:400-407. DOI: 10.1007/s11999.0000000000000012

[153] Tírico LEP, Pasqualin T, Pécora JO, Gobbi RG, Pécora JR, Demange MK. Estudo da estabilidade dos componentes na artroplastia total do joelho sem cimento. Acta Ortopédica Brasileira. 2012;**20**(4):230-234. DOI: 10.1590/s1413-78522012000400008

[154] Fraser JF, Werner S, Jacofsky DJ. Wear and loosening in total knee

arthroplasty: A quick review. The Journal of Knee Surgery. 2015;**28**:139-144. DOI: 10.1055/s-0034-1398375

[155] Naudie DDR, Ammeen DJ, Engh GA, Rorabeck CH. Wear and osteolysis around total knee arthroplasty. The Journal of the American Academy of Orthopaedic Surgeons. 2007;**15**:53-64

[156] Bozic KJ, Kurtz SM, Lau E, Ong K, Chiu V, Vail TP, et al. The epidemiology of revision total knee arthroplasty in the United States. Clinical Orthopaedics and Related Research. 2010;**468**:45-51. DOI: 10.1007/s11999-009-0945-0

[157] Peters PC, Engh GA, Dwyer KA, Vinh TN. Osteolysis after total knee arthroplasty without cement. The Journal of Bone and Joint Surgery. American Volume. 1992;**74**:864-876

[158] Robinson EJ, Mulliken BD, Bourne RB, Rorabeck CH, Alvarez C. Catastrophic osteolysis in total knee replacement. A report of 17 cases. Clinical Orthopaedics and Related Research. 1995;**321**:98-105

[159] Callaghan JJ, O'Rourke MR, Liu SS. The role of implant constraint in revision total knee arthroplasty: Not too little, not too much. Journal of Arthroplasty. 2005;**20**:41-43

[160] Doolittle KH, Turner RH. Patellofemoral problems following total knee arthroplasty. Orthopaedic Review. 1988;**17**:696-702

[161] Bozic KJ, Kamath AF, Ong K, Lau E, Kurtz S, Chan V, et al. Comparative epidemiology of revision arthroplasty: Failed THA poses greater clinical and economic burdens than failed TKA. Clinical Orthopaedics and Related Research. 2015;**473**:2131-2138. DOI: 10.1007/s11999-014-4078-8

[162] Vince KG. The problem total knee replacement: Systematic, comprehensive and efficient evaluation. The The Bone and Joint Journal 2014;96-B:105-111. doi:10.1302/0301-620X.96B11.34531

[163] Doolittle KH, Turner RH. Patellofemoral problems following total knee arthroplasty. Orthopaedic Review. 1988

[164] Young SW, Saffi M, Spangehl MJ, Clarke HD. Unexplained pain following total knee arthroplasty: Is rotational malalignment the problem? The Knee. 2018. DOI: 10.1016/j.knee.2018.01.011

[165] Czurda T, Fennema P, Baumgartner M, Ritschl P. The association between component malalignment and post-operative pain following navigation-assisted total knee arthroplasty: Results of a cohort/nested case-control study. The Knee Surgery, Sports Traumatology, Arthroscopy. 2010. DOI: 10.1007/s00167-009-0990-y

[166] Longo UG, Ciuffreda M, Mannering N, D'Andrea V, Cimmino M, Denaro V, et al. Patellar resurfacing in total knee arthroplasty: Systematic review and meta-analysis. Journal of Arthroplasty. 2017. DOI:10.1016/j.arth.2017.08.041 LK. Available from: http://sfxit.ugent.be/ugent?sid=EMBASE&issn=15328406&id=doi:10.1016%2Fj.arth.2017.08.041&atitle=Patellar+Resurfacing+in+Total+Knee+Arthroplasty%3A+Systematic+Review+and+Meta-Analysis&stitle=J.+Arthroplasty&title=Journal+of+Arthroplasty&volume=&issue=&spage=&epage=&aulast=Longo&aufirst=Umile+G.&auinit=U.G.&aufull=Longo+U.G.&coden=JOARE&isbn=&pages=-&date=2017&auinit-1=U&auinitm=G

[167] Petersen W, Rembitzki IV, Brüggemann GP, Ellermann A, Best R, Koppenburg AG, et al. Anterior knee pain after total knee arthroplasty: A narrative review. International Orthopaedics. 2014;**38**(2):319-328. DOI: 10.1007/s00264-013-2081-4

Chapter 6

Stiffness after Primary Total Knee Arthroplasty

Vishavpreet Singh, Galen Berdis, Akshay Goel, Alisina Shahi and Ali Oliashirazi

Abstract

Total knee arthroplasty remains the definitive treatment for end-stage osteoarthritis of the knee. Despite being a very successful intervention in terms of relieving pain and returning a patient's function, it is not without complications. Post-operative stiffness after total knee arthroplasty is one of those complications that can be puzzling for physicians and debilitating for patients. While the etiology of stiffness is multifactorial, the treatment options are essentially limited to manipulation under anesthesia, removal of adhesions and revision total knee arthroplasty. With patient outcomes directly related to relief of pain and post-operative range of motion, it is paramount that surgeons do all that is necessary to minimize risk of post-operative stiffness.

Keywords: total knee arthroplasty, stiffness, manipulation under anesthesia, revision total knee arthroplasty

1. Introduction

Total knee arthroplasty (TKA) remains the mainstay of treatment in terms of pain relief, restoring mobility, and quality of life improvement for patients with end-stage osteoarthritis of the knee. Pain relief and postoperative range of motion (ROM) have consistently been the two variables of most importance to patients [1–3]. Stiffness after TKA can be debilitating due to pain and functional limitations in daily activities such as going up or down the stairs and sitting or arising from a chair. This chapter discusses the prevalence, etiology, and management of stiffness after primary TKA.

2. Prevalence

The reported incidence of stiffness after TKA varies greatly in literature with rates ranging from 1.3 to 12% [4, 5]. This wide range of incidence results largely due to lack of a consistent widely accepted definition of stiffness after TKA. Laubenthal et al. reported in their quantitative analysis of knee range of motion during activities of daily living (ADL) that patients required a mean of 83 degrees of knee flexion to climb stairs, 93 degrees to sit in a chair without using their hands and 106 degrees for tying their shoes while seated [6]. In fact, many authors use a cut-off of around 95 degrees of flexion to define stiffness as that allows patients to do most of their ADLs [7]. What is less clear is perhaps, at what time point in the postoperative period must a patient obtain 95° [7–9]. Based on the international consensus definition for stiffness according to restriction in ROM, the severity may be graded according to loss of movement based on the deviation from full flexion or extension as mild, moderate, and severe extension restriction (5–10, 11–20, >20) or flexion range (90–100, 70–89, <70) [10]. However, no consensus statement was made on time frame.

3. Etiology

The etiology of stiffness is multifactorial and the associated risk factors can be evaluated by dividing them into three categories: preoperative, intraoperative, and postoperative.

3.1 Preoperative risk factors

There are several preoperative risk factors that may contribute to stiffness after TKA and can be further subcategorized into modifiable versus nonmodifiable.

3.1.1 Modifiable

The major modifiable risk factor is preoperative ROM. Preoperative ROM has consistently been shown to be one of the best predictors of postoperative ROM. Patients with decreased preoperative ROM often have decreased postoperative ROM as well as lower functional scores compared to those without decreased preoperative ROM [11, 12]. With respect to flexion, studies have shown that patients with poor preoperative flexion (<90 degrees) tend to gain flexion postoperatively and those with good preoperative flexion (>105 degrees) experience a net loss in flexion, yet retain a greater ROM overall [13, 14].

3.1.2 Nonmodifiable

Certain patients, that senior author calls "scar-formers", may be at increased risk of stiffness due to their genetic makeup. Several studies have implicated the role of genetics in the formation of arthrofibrosis [15, 16]. It is unclear how to identify these Scar-formers as literature is lacking on whether or not patients with previous keloids or hypertrophic scars go onto to develop stiffness after TKA. At the very least, these findings may serve as a reminder to the treating physician to pay particular attention to these patients as they progress through their postoperative rehabilitation.

While a history of previous surgery and/or trauma has certainly been shown to adversely influence outcomes after TKA, whether or not previous surgery predicts postoperative ROM or stiffness is less clear [17]. In a study by Scranton et al., 85% of the patients with a stiff knee after TKA had previous surgery or diabetes mellitus [9]. Another study evaluating the results of total knee arthroplasty after failed proximal tibial osteotomy for osteoarthritis, reported average arc of motion to be 8 degrees less in TKA patients with prior history of failed proximal tibial osteotomy than those without it. Despite the small difference in arc of motion, the final average arc of motion was 95 degrees in the osteotomy group and there were no differences in rate of people undergoing manipulation for stiffness when compared to those without the osteotomy [18]. Similarly, Harvey et al. showed previous proximal tibial osteotomy had no effect on ultimate ROM [13]. Patients that underwent TKA after a failed unicompartmental knee arthroplasty have demonstrated mean postoperative arcs of motion between 104 and 115 degrees [19]. When comparing patients undergoing TKA for primary osteoarthritis versus post-traumatic osteoarthritis, literature demonstrates that overall there is significant improvement in postoperative ROM when compared to preoperative ROM in both cohorts [20, 21]. However, the improvements were significantly inferior in the post-traumatic cohort [20]. Ultimately, we suspect that the specific type of prior surgery and/or trauma may play a significant role in determining its effect on postoperative ROM.

Lastly, obesity itself has not been shown to be a significant risk factor for postoperative stiffness, but patients with large thigh diameters may have reduced range of motion with flexion due to a mechanical block from abutment of soft tissues [22].

3.2 Intraoperative risk factors

Total knee arthroplasty should be thought of as a patient-specific procedure. Each patient's anatomy and deformity presents a unique challenge and no two consecutive knee arthroplasties are the same and therefore, attention to small details is crucial for a successful result. Most of the intraoperative variables that contribute to postoperative stiffness are related to the surgical technique. Improper gap balancing, incorrect component sizing or positioning, excessively elevating or lowering the joint line, incomplete resection of osteophytes, and closure techniques can all contribute to stiffness in both flexion and extension.

Improper gap balancing can lead to a joint that is "overstuffed" in flexion and/or extension, resulting in a stiff joint. Gap balancing can be easily understood by applying McPherson rules: if the tightness is symmetric in both flexion and extension, problem lies in the proximal tibia resection and if the tightness is asymmetric (i.e. tight in flexion but not in extension and vice versa), problem lies in the femoral resection. Excessive tightness in extension is caused by inadequate distal femur resection, tight posterior capsule, and inadequate resection of osteophytes. If tightness is present in both flexion and extension, it is generally due to a polyethylene insert that is too thick or insufficient proximal tibial resection. Excessive tightness in flexion is often caused by inadequate posterior femoral cut, decreased tibial slope, an oversized femoral component, and a femoral component that is shift posteriorly or malrotated. If using a cruciate retaining implant, a tight posterior cruciate ligament can also limit flexion. Furthermore, intimate knowledge of the instrumentation used during TKA is crucial as when an anterior referencing guide is used, the selection of a larger femoral component leads to tightness in flexion if sizing guide measurement is in between sizes.

While gap balancing in the sagittal plane is important, the patellofemoral joint (PFJ) deserves equal attention as overstuffing the PFJ can lead to tightness of the extensor mechanism and stiffness after TKA. PFJ is usually overstuffed due to two reasons: (i) inadequate resection of the patella or (ii) anterior placement of the femoral component. Generally speaking, the amount of patellar bone resected should equal the width of the patellar component while also keeping in mind the thickness of the cartilage that may not be present at the time of TKA. In a study by Alcerro et al., patients in whom the patellar thickness after TKA was restored as close to the native thickness demonstrated the greatest improvements in quality of life, physical measures and Western Ontario and McMaster Universities Arthritis Index stiffness scores [23].

Additionally, their study also showed that patients who reported more stiffness and lower knee active flexion had greater than native patella thickness after surgery [23]. Studies by Daluga et al. and Shoji et al. further show that an increase of 12% in anterior–posterior diameter of the knee and increase of 20% in patellar thickness, respectively, leads to marked increase in postoperative stiffness [8, 22]. In a similar fashion, joint line elevation can lead to issues with PFJ kinematics and cause stiffness after TKA. Elevated joint line, whether due to inadequate resection of tibia, excessive resection of distal femur, or thick polyethylene inserts, leads to patella baja. Patella baja has been associated with decreased postoperative ROM and patient reported outcome measures [24, 25]. The importance of maintaining correct patellar height is further demonstrated by Vives-Barquiel et al. by showing improvements in flexion and clinical scores after osteotomy of the tibial tuberosity to move it proximally in knees with postoperative patella baja [26]. Of course, there is potential for catastrophic complication with this procedure, including nonunion and escape.

Lastly, several studies have demonstrated that knee position (i.e. flexion, semi-flexed, versus extended) during surgical wound closure may influence postoperative ROM. In a literature review by Faour et al., authors concluded that wound closure in flexion was associated with significant improvement in ROM recovery at earlier follow-ups after TKA and faster physical recovery compared with wound closure in extension. However, no difference was noticed in long-term ROM recovery when comparing closure with knee in flexion versus extension [27]. On the contrary, studies by Motififard et al. and Masri et al. demonstrated no differences in postoperative ROM with knees closed in flexion versus extension [28, 29].

3.3 Postoperative risk factors

Postoperative risk factors that can contribute to stiffness include lack of patient participation/compliance with therapy, uncontrolled pain, complex regional pain syndrome (CRPS), heterotrophic ossification (HO), infection, patellar complications, and arthrofibrosis. Postoperative physical therapy is an integral component of recovery after TKA, as patients often have issues with gait, balance, strength, and ROM. It requires significant commitment on the part of the both the physician and the patient to come up with an individualized plan meet postoperative rehabilitation goals. Poorly motivated patients are less likely to mobilize after surgery, comply with postoperative ROM and more likely to have a prolonged hospital stay. It is pertinent to identify these patients early (often even before surgery) and intervene early.

Uncontrolled pain or CRPS can also prohibit patients from exerting their maximum effort at therapy and must be correctly identified early and correct interventions including a possible referral to pain management be instituted. The incidence of postoperative infection after TKA is around 2% and should be considered in any patient with postoperative stiffness. If suspicion for infection is high appropriate labs including ESR, CRP and possible aspiration must be obtained to rule out an infection. Patellar complications such as unresurfaced patella, avascular necrosis of patella, patellar fracture, or mal-tracking can also cause also cause pain and stiffness. Lastly, while the incidence of radiographic HO after TKA may be as high as 26%, it is rare to find HO significant enough to limit ROM.

4. Management

The most important aspect of management for a stiff TKA is identifying the underlying etiology.

There are several treatment options available for stiffness after TKA including observation with more aggressive physical therapy, manipulation under anesthesia (MUA), surgical debridement, and revision total knee arthroplasty (rTKA). All of these strategies are only successful if done for the right indications. For example, a patient with stiff knee due to component misalignment or underlying infection is not likely to respond to a MUA.

4.1 Manipulation under anesthesia (MUA)

MUA should be considered when stiffness persists despite an aggressive program to gain motion.

Since MUA is not a benign procedure given the risk of fracture, extensor mechanism disruption, and hemarthrosis, correct patient selection is crucial. Anterior femoral notching is considered an absolute contraindication to MUA due to increased risk of femoral fractures. When it comes to MUA, one is faced with two questions: (i) which patients to manipulate? And (ii) what is the best time for manipulation? The answer to the first question lies in how one defines post-operative stiffness. Some physicians may stick to a strict number (i.e. flexion <90 by 6 weeks) and offer to manipulate everyone who fails to meet those criteria. However, the issue with a strict-number definition of TKA is that a patient who may not be considered to have stiffness (based on the aforementioned criteria, for example) might in fact be the one who needs the MUA as his/her activity requirements may consist of kneeling and hence greater need for flexion, as is often the case in Middle Eastern cultures. Therefore, the decision to proceed with a TKA should be centered on a joint conversation between the patient and the physician. We have patients in our practice who are very content with a ROM of 0–85 degrees, as they are able to do all the activities that they desire to do and therefore, do not need a MUA.

With respect to the timing for MUA, there is no consensus in the literature. Studies demonstrate both increased and no additional benefit with early MUA. In their review of patients undergoing MUA for stiffness, Issa et al. report that patients who underwent early MUA (<12 weeks postoperatively) had significantly higher mean gain in flexion (36.5 versus 17), higher final range of motion (119 versus 95 degrees) and higher function scores (88 versus 83) than those who had late (>12 weeks postoperatively) MUA [30]. Furthermore, when they sub-stratified outcomes based incremental time to MUA demonstrated that there was significant drop in range of motion gained after MUA as more time elapsed postoperatively. While some range of motion was gained with MUA at all periods postoperatively, authors reported that best results were obtained when MUA was done within 12 weeks postoperatively and significantly worse at 26 weeks (36.5 versus 12 degrees). Other authors who found higher gains in flexion with early MUA reported similar results [7, 22, 31–33]. Yercan et al. reported a study of 46 patients that underwent MUA for stiffness after TKA had mean flexion arc improvement from 67+/−11 to 114+/−16 degrees. Furthermore, patients that underwent a MUA within the first 3 weeks after TKA had significantly higher final range of motion compared with those who underwent after 3 months (121+/−11 versus 112+/−16). Similarly, Namba et al. reported that although both early and late MUA result in significant gains in flexion arc, early manipulation resulted in approximately twice the mean flexion gains [31].

In contrast to the above studies, there are several studies that have shown no difference in outcomes when stratified based on timing of MUA. Yeoh et al. report on 48 patients that underwent MUA for stiffness and they noticed that at 1 year there was no difference in gain in ROM between knees that were manipulated within 12 weeks postoperatively versus after 12 weeks [34]. Similarly, Keating et al. report their results of 113 MUAs in 90 patients followed for a mean of 4.6 years and noticed that mean knee flexion improved from 70 to 105 degrees, however, no significant difference was found for patients that underwent MUA before or after 12 weeks after TKA ($p = 0.36$) [35].

4.2 Surgical treatment

Surgical treatment of stiffness in the forms of arthroscopic or open lysis of adhesions with or without MUA after TKA should be considered as the last resort after a patient has failed both physical therapy and MUA (or is outside the time window where MUA alone might not be beneficial). While arthroscopic debridement of adhesions with MUA has shown promising results in patients with stiffness from procedures other than TKA, this is not always the case for patients who have it done after TKA [36–39]. Campbell reports an increase of only 11 degrees in flexion and 55 degrees in extension for 8 patients in 1 year after arthroscopy. Similarly, Bocell et al. report that only 2 out of 7 patients maintained pain-free improvements in ROM after arthroscopic debridement and MUA after TKA. On the contrary, other authors have reported marked improvements in ROM after arthroscopic lysis. Tjoumakaris et al. report in their study that after arthroscopic lysis with gentle manipulation for stiffness after TKA, mean flexion improved from 79 to 103 degrees and mean extension deficit from 16 to 4 degrees at average of 31 months, leading authors to conclude that arthroscopic lysis of adhesions is a reliable procedure [40]. However, they also noticed that patients achieved approximately half of the improvement that was obtained at the time of surgery. Volchenko et al. report on a matched cohort study of 35 patients treated with MUA and 35 patients treated with arthroscopic lysis of adhesions plus MUA. Arthroscopic lysis with MUA yielded changes in ROM: a 72.7% increase 4 to 12 weeks after index TKA ($p = 0.032$), a 50.0% increase 12+ weeks after TKA ($p = 0.032$), and a 99.8% increase in patients with a pre-manipulation ROM of 0–60 degrees ($p = 0.001$). MUA alone yielded a 49.2% increase 4 to 12 weeks after index TKA ($p = 0.161$), a 27.0% increase 12+ weeks after TKA ($p = 0.161$) and a 68.8% increase in patients with pre-manipulation ROM of 0 to 60 degrees [41]. Authors concluded arthroscopic lysis of adhesions plus MUA led to greater increases in ROM ($p = 0.026$) and final knee flexion ($p = 0.028$) compare with those treated with MUA alone. After arthroscopic lysis of adhesions and manipulation, Diduch et al., Scranton, and Bae et al. also report similar results with mean flexion improvement of 26 degrees, mean gain in ROM of 31 degrees, and mean improvement in arc of motion of 42 degrees, respectively [9, 42, 43]. There is evidence in literature that for patients with a PCL-retaining implant and limitations in ROM (especially flexion), there may be a benefit from arthroscopic release of PCL. Williams et al. report a mean flexion increase of 30 degrees and mean extension improvement from 4 to 1.5 degrees at 20 month follow up 10 knees after arthroscopic release of PCL.

Lastly, revision TKA should be reserved for patients when a clear diagnosis for the cause of stiffness (i.e. malpositioning of components, infection, loosening, etc.) can be made and corrected during surgery as these patients have more predictable results compared to revisions done in patients without a clear-cut diagnosis [44–47]. Hartman et al. report on 35 patients that underwent rTKA for stiffness and at mean of 54.5 months, the mean arc of motion improved by 44.5 degrees. However, 49% (17/35) of the patients required a further intervention for stiffness or sustained a complication. Authors concluded that while rTKA can be performed with reasonable expectation of improvement in ROM, the complication risk is significant [48]. Ries et al. reported better results with rTKA in 6 knees with mean increase in arc of motion of 50 degrees at minimum of 2 year follow up for patients with stiffness secondary to arthrofibrosis only [49]. Generally, results of rTKA specifically for stiffness are less predictable and may be influenced by surgical technique and patient's response to surgical trauma.

5. Conclusion

TKA is an excellent option for patients with end-stage knee osteoarthritis in terms of pain relief. Postoperative stiffness continues to be a challenge for both the physicians and the patients. Due to the multifactorial etiology of stiffness, the interventions to address it are limited to MUA, lysis of adhesions, and revision TKA. The results with each intervention are variable, especially with surgical options.

Author details

Vishavpreet Singh[1], Galen Berdis[1], Akshay Goel[1], Alisina Shahi[2*]
and Ali Oliashirazi[1]

1 Oliashirazi Institute at Marshall University, Huntington, West Virginia, USA

2 Cooper Bone and Joint Institute at Cooper Medical School of Rowan University, Camden, NJ, USA

*Address all correspondence to: alisinair@gmail.com

References

[1] Bourne RB, Chesworth BM, Davis AM, Mahomed NN, Charron KDJ. Patient satisfaction after total knee arthroplasty: Who is satisfied and who is not? Clinical Orthopaedics and Related Research. 2010;**468**(1):57-63. DOI: 10.1007/s11999-009-1119-9

[2] Matsuda S, Kawahara S, Okazaki K, Tashiro Y, Iwamoto Y. Postoperative alignment and ROM affect patient satisfaction after TKA. Clinical Orthopaedics and Related Research. 2013;**471**(1):127-133. DOI: 10.1007/s11999-012-2533-y

[3] Williams DP, O'Brien S, Doran E, et al. Early postoperative predictors of satisfaction following total knee arthroplasty. The Knee. 2013;**20**(6):442-446. DOI: 10.1016/j.knee.2013.05.011

[4] Bong MR, Di Cesare PE. Stiffness after total knee arthroplasty. The Journal of the American Academy of Orthopaedic Surgeons. 2004;**12**(3):164-171

[5] Parvizi J, Tarity TD, Steinbeck MJ, et al. Management of stiffness following total knee arthroplasty. The Journal of Bone and Joint Surgery. American Volume. 2006;**88**(Suppl 4):175-181. DOI: 10.2106/JBJS.F.00608

[6] Laubenthal KN, Smidt GL, Kettelkamp DB. A quantitative analysis of knee motion during activities of daily living. Physical Therapy. 1972;**52**(1):34-43. DOI: 10.1093/ptj/52.1.34

[7] Yercan HS, Sugun TS, Bussiere C, Ait Si Selmi T, Davies A, Neyret P. Stiffness after total knee arthroplasty: Prevalence, management and outcomes. The Knee. 2006;**13**(2):111-117. DOI: 10.1016/j.knee.2005.10.001

[8] Shoji H, Solomonow M, Yoshino S, D'Ambrosia R, Dabezies E. Factors affecting postoperative flexion in total knee arthroplasty. Orthopedics. 1990;**13**(6):643-649

[9] Scranton PE. Management of knee pain and stiffness after total knee arthroplasty. The Journal of Arthroplasty. 2001;**16**(4):428-435. DOI: 10.1054/arth.2001.22250

[10] Kalson NS, Borthwick LA, Mann DA, et al. International consensus on the definition and classification of fibrosis of the knee joint. The Bone & Joint Journal. 2016;**98-B**(11):1479-1488. DOI: 10.1302/0301-620X.98B10.37957

[11] Shi M, Lü H, Guan Z. Influence of preoperative range of motion on the early clinical outcome of total knee arthroplasty. Zhonghua Wai Ke Za Zhi. 2006;**44**(16):1101-1105

[12] Ritter MA, Harty LD, Davis KE, Meding JB, Berend ME. Predicting range of motion after total knee arthroplasty. Clustering, log-linear regression, and regression tree analysis. The Journal of Bone and Joint Surgery. American Volume. 2003;**85**(7):1278-1285. DOI: 10.2106/00004623-200307000-00014

[13] Harvey IA, Barry K, Kirby SP, Johnson R, Elloy MA. Factors affecting the range of movement of total knee arthroplasty. Journal of Bone and Joint Surgery. British Volume (London). 1993;**75**(6):950-955

[14] Parsley BS, Engh GA, Dwyer KA. Preoperative flexion. Does it influence postoperative flexion after posterior-cruciate-retaining total knee arthroplasty? Clinical Orthopaedics and Related Research. 1992;**275**:204-210

[15] Hakim AJ, Cherkas LF, Spector TD, MacGregor AJ. Genetic associations between frozen shoulder and tennis elbow: A female twin

study. Rheumatology (Oxford). 2003;**42**(6):739-742. DOI: 10.1093/rheumatology/keg159

[16] Usher KM, Zhu S, Mavropalias G, Carrino JA, Zhao J, Xu J. Pathological mechanisms and therapeutic outlooks for arthrofibrosis. Bone Research. 2019;7:9. DOI: 10.1038/s41413-019-0047-x

[17] Steinhoff AK, Bugbee WD. Outcomes of total knee arthroplasty after osteochondral allograft transplantation. Orthopaedic Journal of Sports Medicine. 2014;**2**(9):2325967114550276. DOI: 10.1177/2325967114550276

[18] Katz MM, Hungerford DS, Krackow KA, Lennox DW. Results of total knee arthroplasty after failed proximal tibial osteotomy for osteoarthritis. The Journal of Bone and Joint Surgery. American Volume. 1987;**69**(2):225-233

[19] Levine WN, Ozuna RM, Scott RD, Thornhill TS. Conversion of failed modern unicompartmental arthroplasty to total knee arthroplasty. The Journal of Arthroplasty. 1996;**11**(7):797-801

[20] Lunebourg A, Parratte S, Gay A, Ollivier M, Garcia-Parra K, Argenson J-N. Lower function, quality of life, and survival rate after total knee arthroplasty for posttraumatic arthritis than for primary arthritis. Acta Orthopaedica. 2015;**86**(2):189-194. DOI: 10.3109/17453674.2014.979723

[21] Saleh H, Yu S, Vigdorchik J, Schwarzkopf R. Total knee arthroplasty for treatment of post-traumatic arthritis: Systematic review. World Journal of Orthopedics. 2016;7(9):584-591. DOI: 10.5312/wjo.v7.i9.584

[22] Daluga D, Lombardi AV, Mallory TH, Vaughn BK. Knee manipulation following total knee arthroplasty. Analysis of prognostic variables. The Journal of Arthroplasty. 1991;**6**(2):119-128

[23] Alcerro JC, Rossi MD, Lavernia CJ. Primary total knee Arthroplasty: How does residual patellar thickness affect patient-oriented outcomes? The Journal of Arthroplasty. 2017;**32**(12):3621-3625. DOI: 10.1016/j.arth.2017.06.046

[24] Behrend H, Graulich T, Gerlach R, Spross C, Ladurner A. Blackburne-Peel ratio predicts patients' outcomes after total knee arthroplasty. Knee Surgery, Sports Traumatology, Arthroscopy. 2019;**27**(5):1562-1569. DOI: 10.1007/s00167-018-5016-1

[25] Figgie HE, Goldberg VM, Heiple KG, Moller HS, Gordon NH. The influence of tibial-patellofemoral location on function of the knee in patients with the posterior stabilized condylar knee prosthesis. The Journal of Bone and Joint Surgery. American Volume. 1986;**68**(7):1035-1040

[26] Vives-Barquiel MA, Torrents A, Lozano L, et al. Proximalize osteotomy of tibial tuberosity (POTT) as a treatment for stiffness secondary to patella Baja in total knee arthroplasty (TKA). Archives of Orthopaedic and Trauma Surgery. 2015;**135**(10):1445-1451. DOI: 10.1007/s00402-015-2312-9

[27] Faour M, Sodhi N, Khlopas A, et al. Knee position during surgical wound closure in total knee arthroplasty: A review. The Journal of Knee Surgery. 2018;**31**(1):6-12. DOI: 10.1055/s-0037-1608838

[28] Motififard M, Heidari M, Nemati A. No difference between wound closure in extension or flexion for range of motion following total knee arthroplasty: A randomized clinical trial. Knee Surgery, Sports Traumatology, Arthroscopy. 2016;**24**(1):74-78. DOI: 10.1007/s00167-014-3317-6

[29] Masri BA, Laskin RS, Windsor RE, Haas SB. Knee closure in total knee replacement: A randomized prospective trial. Clinical Orthopaedics and Related Research. 1996;**331**:81-86. DOI: 10.1097/00003086-199610000-00011

[30] Issa K, Banerjee S, Kester MA, Khanuja HS, Delanois RE, Mont MA. The effect of timing of manipulation under anesthesia to improve range of motion and functional outcomes following total knee arthroplasty. The Journal of Bone and Joint Surgery. American Volume. 2014;**96**(16):1349-1357. DOI: 10.2106/JBJS.M.00899

[31] Namba RS, Inacio M. Early and late manipulation improve flexion after total knee arthroplasty. The Journal of Arthroplasty. 2007;**22**(6 Suppl 2):58-61. DOI: 10.1016/j.arth.2007.02.010

[32] Fitzsimmons SE, Vazquez EA, Bronson MJ. How to treat the stiff total knee arthroplasty?: A systematic review. Clinical Orthopaedics and Related Research. 2010;**468**(4):1096-1106. DOI: 10.1007/s11999-010-1230-y

[33] Esler CN, Lock K, Harper WM, Gregg PJ. Manipulation of total knee replacements. Is the flexion gained retained? Journal of Bone and Joint Surgery. British Volume (London). 1999;**81**(1):27-29

[34] Yeoh D, Nicolaou N, Goddard R, et al. Manipulation under anaesthesia post total knee replacement: Long term follow up. The Knee. 2012;**19**(4):329-331. DOI: 10.1016/j.knee.2011.05.009

[35] Keating EM, Ritter MA, Harty LD, et al. Manipulation after total knee arthroplasty. The Journal of Bone and Joint Surgery. American Volume. 2007;**89**(2):282-286. DOI: 10.2106/JBJS.E.00205

[36] Sprague NF. Motion-limiting arthrofibrosis of the knee: The role of arthroscopic management. Clinics in Sports Medicine. 1987;**6**(3):537-549

[37] Sprague NF, O'Connor RL, Fox JM. Arthroscopic treatment of postoperative knee fibroarthrosis. Clinical Orthopaedics and Related Research. 1982;**166**:165-172

[38] Campbell ED. Arthroscopy in total knee replacements. Arthroscopy. 1987;**3**(1):31-35

[39] Bocell JR, Thorpe CD, Tullos HS. Arthroscopic treatment of symptomatic total knee arthroplasty. Clinical Orthopaedics and Related Research. 1991;**271**:125-134

[40] Tjoumakaris FP, Tucker BC, Post Z, Pepe MD, Orozco F, Ong AC. Arthroscopic lysis of adhesions for the stiff total knee: Results after failed manipulation. Orthopedics. 2014;**37**(5):e482-e487. DOI: 10.3928/01477447-20140430-60

[41] Volchenko E, Schwarzman G, Robinson M, Chmell SJ, Gonzalez MH. Arthroscopic Lysis of adhesions with manipulation under anesthesia versus manipulation alone in the treatment of arthrofibrosis after TKA: A matched cohort study. Orthopedics. 2019;**42**(3):163-167. DOI: 10.3928/01477447-20190424-08

[42] Diduch DR, Scuderi GR, Scott WN, Insall JN, Kelly MA. The efficacy of arthroscopy following total knee replacement. Arthroscopy. 1997;**13**(2):166-171

[43] Bae DK, Lee HK, Cho JH. Arthroscopy of symptomatic total knee replacements. Arthroscopy. 1995;**11**(6):664-671

[44] Babis GC, Trousdale RT, Pagnano MW, Morrey BF. Poor outcomes of isolated tibial insert exchange and arthrolysis for the management

of stiffness following total knee arthroplasty. The Journal of Bone and Joint Surgery. American Volume. 2001;**83**(10):1534-1536. DOI: 10.2106/00004623-200110000-00012

[45] Ritter MA, Stringer EA. Predictive range of motion after total knee replacement. Clinical Orthopaedics and Related Research. 1979;**143**:115-119

[46] Haidukewych GJ, Jacofsky DJ, Pagnano MW, Trousdale RT. Functional results after revision of well-fixed components for stiffness after primary total knee arthroplasty. The Journal of Arthroplasty. 2005;**20**(2):133-138

[47] Nicholls DW, Dorr LD. Revision surgery for stiff total knee arthroplasty. The Journal of Arthroplasty. 1990;**5**(Suppl):S73-S77

[48] Hartman CW, Ting NT, Moric M, Berger RA, Rosenberg AG, Della Valle CJ. Revision total knee arthroplasty for stiffness. The Journal of Arthroplasty. 2010;**25**(6 Suppl):62-66. DOI: 10.1016/j.arth.2010.04.013

[49] Ries MD, Badalamente M. Arthrofibrosis after total knee arthroplasty. Clinical Orthopaedics and Related Research. 2000;**380**:177-183. DOI: 10.1097/00003086-200011000-00024

Chapter 7

Management of Flexion Contracture in Total Knee Arthroplasty

Kavin Khatri, Deepak Bansal and Karan Rajpal

Abstract

Fixed flexion deformity at knee is common in osteoarthritic knee and is a combination of bony deformity, capsular and ligamentous deformity. It affects knee biomechanics in terms of increased forces at the patellofemoral and tibiofemoral joint. This in turn makes carrying out of routine daily activities like walking or use of staircase very difficult. Therefore, it is essential to correct this deformity at the time of operative intervention. Major interventions like posterior capsular release and removal of osteophytes and adequate bony resection helps in correcting the deformity. Post operatively, use of extension night splints and adequate physiotherapy can help in correcting the residual deformity left over at the time of knee arthroplasty.

Keywords: total knee arthroplasty, fixed flexion deformity, range of motion, flexion contracture

1. Introduction

Flexion deformity at knee in osteoarthritis or rheumatoid arthritis is due to synovial inflammation leading to fluid in joint subsequently resulting in assuming of position maximum accommodation i.e. flexion. Posterior femoral and tibal osteophytes tent upon the capsule resulting in further flexion at the knee and sometimes mechanical block to extension. Other factors like hamstring shortening and ligament contracture also contribute to flexion at the knee. There is increase in energy expenditure while walking or standing along with decreased endurance and inability to stand for long period of time [1–2]. Fixed flexion at single knee increases abnormal forces on other knee resulting in abnormal gait. There is limb length discrepancy and short stride length. There is associated increase in extension and adduction. In severe flexion deformities, there is alteration of kinematics of spine. There are increased chances of lumbar spondylosis and accelerated degeneration of contralateral knee in cases of long standing flexion deformity at knee. Isolated flexion deformity is very rare and generally associated with either varus or valgus deformity at knee [3]. Some authors have reported incidence of flexion deformity up to 60° in cases of osteoarthritis knee [4]. To achieve complete range of movement at knee, full surgical correction should be achieved during surgical correction.

2. Prevalence and risk factors

Ritter et al. [5] had described that residual flexion contracture by more than 10 degree can result in poor functional outcome in patients who undergo knee replacement. The risk factors for persistence of deformity were male gender, higher age and preoperative flexion contracture of more than five or more degrees [6]. Among these the single most important factor predictive of residual flexion contracture was preoperative flexion deformity at knee. Body mass index has no role in persistence of flexion deformity after surgical correction [7]. Surgical technique factor like overstuffing of extension gap and flexion of femoral component also determines the post-operative flexion deformity. The femoral component placed in flexion can result in limitation of arc of motion due to constraints in articulation.

3. Pathoanatomy

Long standing cases of arthritis have intercondylar osteophytes, which acts as mechanical block to extension [4]. The posterior osteophytes in addition impinge upon posterior capsule further increasing flexion contracture. Subsequently, it leads to contraction of soft tissues over the posterior aspect of knee adding to the deformity.

There is erosion of the posterior aspect of the tibia and reduction in the strength of quadriceps resulting in extension lag even after correction of deformity. Lombardi et al. [8] had classified flexion deformity into three grades depending upon the severity of deformity. Grade I is mild contracture with deformity limited to less than 15°. Grade II is moderate contracture with deformity between 15° and 30°. Grade III is severe contracture with deformity greater than 30°.

4. Preoperative preparation

A patient with knee flexion contracture undergoing knee replacement should be evaluated for coronal plane deformities, grade of flexion deformity, extensor lag and preoperative range of motion is recorded. The assessment of these variables helps a surgeon to decide regarding the clinical expectations, surgical technique, associated risks and complications. The next important step is to grade the flexion contracture. The standard radiographs should be evaluated to determine the disturbances in the bony anatomy especially posterior condylar deficiencies, coronal deformities and prominent osteophytes. The posterior condylar deficiency affects the rotation of femoral component when posterior referencing system or measured resection technique is used. Sometimes large bony defects would require augments in the form of allografts or modular inserts.

5. Preoperative measures to treat flexion deformity

In patients suffering from inflammatory arthritis, there is minimal or no osteophyte formation associated with fixed flexion deformity hence preoperative manipulation is sometimes helpful in selected cases. In cases with bilateral hip and knee deformity, the preoperative manipulation is carried out after hip replacement with the aid of serial casting over the knee in maximal stretch [9]. The cast should be adequately padded to avoid pressure sores over the anterior aspect of knee. Epidural anesthesia can be very helpful in these cases as serial casting becomes relatively pain free and fruitful.

6. Surgical technique

After all preoperative preparations, tourniquet is applied over the limb to operated and activated just before incision. The operative leg is examined again under anesthesia to ascertain the degree of deformities. Limb is draped and prepared with betadine or chlorhexidine solution as per the hospital infection control protocols. A midline skin incision is given extending approximately 5 cm proximal to suprapatellar pouch to a point just medial to tibial tubercle. Medial parapatellar osteotomy is performed with eversion of patella exposing both lateral and medial femoral condyle. Next step is to correction of coronal deformities with removal of osteophytes and soft tissue contractures. All efforts should be concentrated to correct the flexion deformity intraoperatively while maintaining soft tissue and adequate stability. The classical approach described by Insall [10] is to resect the posterior femoral condyle and releasing the soft tissues in order to achieve a rectangular flexion gap. Another technique of balancing is to measure the resected pieces of bones from femoral and tibial condyle and replacing the same with components of same size.

The primary focus in case of fixed flexion deformity is over the posterior femoral recess. The posterior capsule should be released as far as possible. The posterior capsule release makes the extension gap equivalent to flexion gap. It also avoids excessive resection of distal femur which can lead to elevation of joint line and mid flexion instability there by altering the patellofemoral kinematics.

7. Grade 1 flexion contracture

Tibial and femoral cuts are carried out in usual manner as in primary uncomplicated arthroplasty. The flexion contracture is due to posterior recess and posterior osteophytes indenting upon the capsule. After the bony cuts, the osteophytes can easily be visualized and removed with the help of ¾ inch osteotome (**Figure 1**). A intramedullary rod may be used to elevate the distal femur or lamina spreaders can be used for better visualization of posterior capsule. There is clear dividing line between the osteophytes and femoral condyle. The loose osteophytes can be removed with the help of curette. The posterior obliterated posterior recess can be then be created with osteotome. The osteophytes from posterior aspect of tibia are visible clearly at this stage and can be removed with the help of curette and osteotome. The osteophytes attached to the posterior capsule is pulled forward and removed with the help of electrocautery. In case extension gap is less than flexion

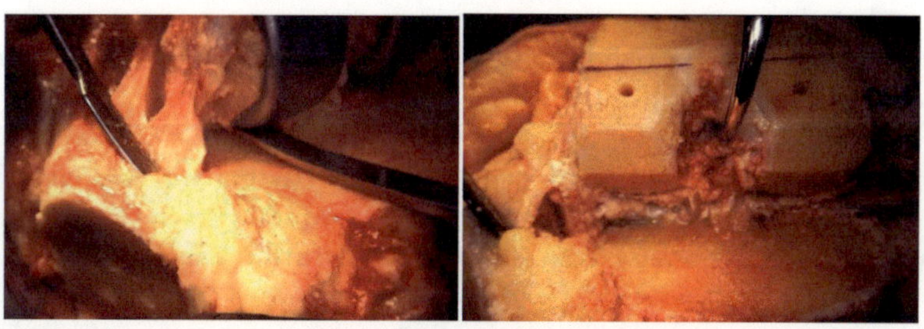

Figure 1.
Posterior osteophytes are removed with the help of osteotome.

gap further release of posterior recess is carried out. However, if extension gap is more than flexion gap, the posterior slope of tibia is evaluated. The slope can be increased up to 8° in order to balance the knee. Tight flexion gap can result in poor roll back of femoral component and lift off of tibia tray.

In majority of the cases, the flexion contracture is corrected with these simple maneuvers. The type of knee prosthesis i.e. cruciate retaining or cruciate sacrificing depends upon the choice of surgeon in mild flexion contracture. Laskin [11] described a test to assess the correction of flexion deformity intraoperatively. The operated limb is lifted from the table and foot is dorsiflexed at ankle subsequently axial pressure is applied along the long axis of the limb. The sudden flexion at knee suggests residual flexion deformity. If there is no bending at knee due to axial pressure then it suggests achievement of adequate correction at the knee joint.

8. Grade II flexion contracture

In addition to release of posterior recess and removal of osteophytes as described in management of grade I flexion, the posterior cruciate ligament is released from the femoral end first and subsequently from the tibial end as per the requirement. Medial and lateral perforations of posterior cruciate ligament can also result in fractional lengthening. With this technique, the cruciate retaining components can be used. In other cases where posterior cruciate ligament is significantly weakened, one should opt for posterior stabilized components.

At the end of all the above releases, if extension gap is smaller than flexion gap, the distal femur is resected by 2 mm. However, if surgeon decides to go ahead with cruciate retaining knee components then distal femur should be resected by more than 4 mm as it can lead to posterior cruciate ligament dysfunction due to elevation of joint line.

9. Grade III flexion contracture

In case of flexion contracture is more than 30°, sequential release is carried out as described in management of grade I and II flexion contracture. The posterior cruciate ligament should be released from its proximal and distal attachment to balance flexion and extension gap at this stage. The choice of implant should preferably be posterior stabilized rather than cruciate retaining. It is important to release posterior capsule and gastrocnemius heads from the posterior aspect of distal femur. In majority of the cases the balanced flexion and extension gap is achieved, however, if there is valgus-varus instability due to laxity of medial or lateral collateral ligament then constrained prosthesis should preferably be used. The lax extensor mechanism can be countered by distal and lateral advancement of vastus medialis and medial capsular structures.

Sequential correction of fixed flexion deformity in total knee replacement (**Figure 2**).

1. Correct coronal deformity with mediolateral balancing and removal of all visible osteophytes. Perform all bony tibial and femoral cuts in the usual manner. In majority of mild flexion contractures, the deformity shall be corrected.

2. The posterior recess should be established with help of osteotome and periosteal elevator. If required the medial and lateral head of gastrocnemius should

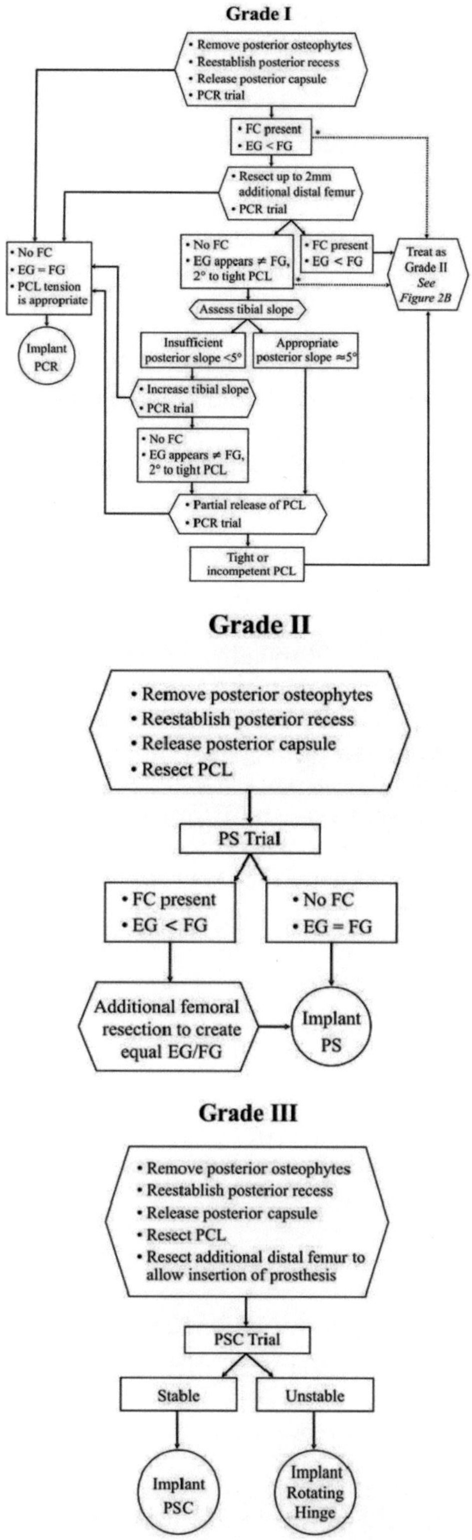

Figure 2.
Treating algorithms for grade I, II and III deformity (EG, extension gap; FC, flexion contracture; FG, flexion gap; PCL, posterior cruciate ligament; PCR, posterior cruciate retaining; PS, posterior stabilized; PSC, posterior stabilized constrained). Reproduced from [12].

also be raised from the posterior and distal end of femur. Sometimes transverse capsulotomy is carried out starting medially and moving laterally. The collaterals are carefully separated from the capsule by longitudinal incisions.

3. In cases of severe flexion deformity, distal femoral resection of up to 4 mm in increments of 2 mm is carried out and gap mismatch is checked. It is advisable to resect minimal bone from the distal femur in order to prevent problem of patellofemoral kinematics, patella baja and elevation of joint line. Sometimes it results in mediolateral instability necessitating the need for constrained prosthesis.

4. Medial and lateral hamstrings are tenotomised in order to achieve full correction in rare cases. Biceps femoris should be clearly identified and separated under vision in order to avoid injury to common peroneal nerve. In cases with flexion deformity of more than 60 degrees, it is advisable to undergo serial casting prior to total knee arthroplasty.

10. Postoperative management

The patients are encouraged to do quadriceps exercises at regular intervals. In cases of mild residual flexion deformity, patients are advised to wear night splints. Stretching exercises play a vital role in the rehabilitation of these cases. It is advised to avoid pillow below the knee and sitting on recliner chairs for a long time as there is tendency towards flexion. The patients should be closely followed in the post-operative period to look for recurrence of deformity. Sometimes patient require manipulation under anesthesia to achieve range of motion similar to that attained in immediate post-operative period. Excessive force should be avoided during manipulation as it might lead to fracture of distal femur.

11. Complications

1. Recurrence of flexion contracture and loss of movement

As stated earlier, the aim should be full correction of flexion deformity intra-operatively. However, at the end of 1 year few cases experience recurrence of deformity.

2. Flexion extension imbalance

Flexion extension instability in case of flexion extension mismatch might require restraint with rotating hinge prostheses.

3. Peroneal nerve injury

Peroneal nerve injury sometimes occurs in cases of fixed flexion with valgus deformity at knee. There could be associated lengthening of the lower limb.

12. Summary

The complexity of surgical procedure increases with increasing flexion deformity of knee. The less complex deformities correct with usual bony resections and removal of osteophytes. Special attention should be paid to creation of posterior capsule. The bony resection especially distal femur should be reserved in cases where soft tissue release achieves inadequate flexion-extension gap match. Postoperatively, the patients should be followed up closely to prevent recurrence of deformity. The patients need monitoring of neurovascular status to miss on an untoward complication.

Author details

Kavin Khatri[1]*, Deepak Bansal[2] and Karan Rajpal[3]

1 Department of Orthopedics, All India Institute of Medical Sciences, Bathinda, Punjab, India

2 AIMC Bassi Hospital, Ludhiana, Punjab, India

3 Department of Orthopedics, GGS Medical College and Hospital, Faridkot, Punjab, India

*Address all correspondence to: kavinkhatri84@gmail.com

References

[1] Harato K, Nagura T, Matsumoto H, Otani T, Toyama Y, Suda Y. Knee fl exion contracture will lead to mechanical overload in both limbs: A simulation study using gait analysis. The Knee. 2008;**15**:467-472

[2] Harato K, Nagura T, Matsumoto H, Otani T, Toyama Y, Suda Y. A gait analysis of simulated knee fl exion contracture to elucidate knee-spine syndrome. Gait & Posture. 2008;**28**:687-692

[3] Su EP. Fixed flexion deformity and total knee arthroplasty. Journal of Bone and Joint Surgery. British Volume (London). 2012;**94**(11 Suppl A):112-115

[4] León HO, Blanco CE, Guthrie TB, Martínez OJ. Intercondylar notch stenosis in degenerative arthritis of the knee. Arthroscopy. 2005;**21**:294-302

[5] Ritter MA, Lutgring JD, Davis KE, et al. The role of flexion contracture on outcomes in primary total knee arthroplasty. The Journal of Arthroplasty. 2007;**22**:1092-1096

[6] Silva A, Tan S, Tay A, Pang HN, Lo NN, Yeo SJ. Risk factors for a postoperative neutrally aligned total knee arthroplasty in the sagittal plane developing fixed flexion deformity at 2 years follow up study. nternational Journal of Research in Orthopaedics. 2019;**5**:211-215

[7] Cheng K, Ridley D, Bird J, McLeod G. Patients with fixed flexion deformity after total knee arthroplasty do just as well as those without: Ten-year prospective data. International Orthopaedics. 2010;**34**(5):663-667. DOI: 10.1007/s00264-009-0801-6

[8] Lombardi AJ, Mallory T, Adams J. A stepwise algorithmic approach to fl exion contractures in total knee arthroplasty. The Journal of the American Academy of Orthopaedic Surgeons. 1997;**1**:1-8

[9] Tateishi H. Contracture of the knee joint. The Journal of Joint Surgery. 1985;**4**:361-365

[10] Insall JN, editor. Surgery of the Knee. New York, NY: Churchill Livingstone; 2000. pp. 1558-1562

[11] Laskin RW, Beksac B. Assess and achieve maximal extension. In: Bellemans J, Ries MD, Victor J, editors. Total Knee Arthroplasty: A Guide to Get Better Performance. Berlin: Springer; 2005. pp. 194-197

[12] Lombard AV Jr, Berend KR. Soft tissue balancing of the knee—Flexion contractures. Techniques in Knee Surgery. 2005;**4**(3):193-206

Chapter 8

Valgus Deformity Correction in Total Knee Replacement: An Overview

Melvin J. George

Abstract

Valgus deformity in total knee replacement is a much lesser encountered problem than varus deformity. The deformity can be caused by either bony or ligamentous pathology or both. Bone defects like lateral cartilage erosion, lateral condylar hypoplasia and metaphyseal femur and tibial plateau remodeling along with soft tissue pathologies like tight lateral collateral ligament (LCL), posterolateral capsule (PLC), popliteus tendon (POP), hamstring tendons, the lateral head of the gastrocnemius (LHG) and iliotibial band (ITB) can add to the magnitude of valgus deformity. Various sequences have been described to achieve balancing while doing a total knee replacement. Proper preoperative planning, clinical examination, necessary implant backup and good operative skill are mandatory to manage bone deformities or soft tissue pathology or both in valgus deformity. Obtaining an accurate axis restoration, component orientation and joint stability in a valgus knee with combined bony and ligamentous pathology may be a difficult task. The long-term results in valgus knees are relatively inferior to those with varus deformity. This chapter structure wise describes the pathology, classification of valgus deformity, radiographic planning, surgical approaches, method of valgus deformity correction, implant selection, associated deformities, precautions and intraoperative complications.

Keywords: valgus, total knee replacement, deformity, balancing, hypoplasia

1. Introduction

Mechanical axis and anatomical axis are the two alignment parameters in the lower extremity. Mechanical axis is the axis or the line of weight bearing through the bone. In the case of straight bone like the tibia, both mechanical and anatomical axes are the same. Mechanical axis of the femur is different from that of anatomical axis. The former is at 5–7° valgus to the anatomical axis (**Figure 1**). Mechanical tibiofemoral angle (1.3 ± 2° varus) or anatomical tibiofemoral angle (6 ± 2° valgus) can be used to denote normal knee joint alignment. Normal mechanical axis of the knee is defined as a line that passes from the centre of the hip to the centre of the ankle. Normal alignment is defined when this line passes through the centre of the knee. A line that falls towards the lateral side of the knee indicates that the lower extremity is in valgus. Varus alignment is more common in males than in females. Valgus deformity is usually defined when the anatomical tibiofemoral angle is equal to or greater than 10°. Since the weight-bearing axis of the lower limb follows

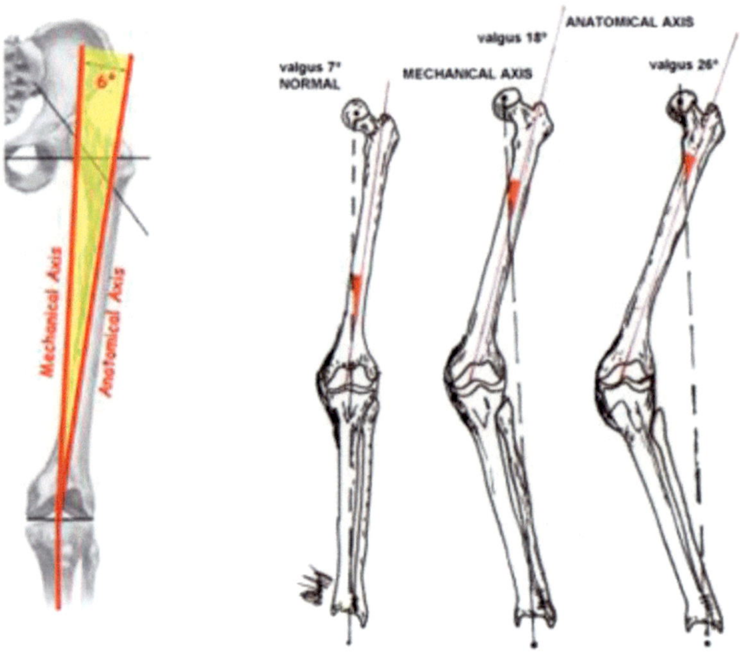

Figure 1.
The method of measuring valgus angle at the knee.

the mechanical axis, a valgus alignment will increase the load in the lateral compartment of the knee. According to Paley and Tetsworth [1], the knee joint is not perpendicular to the mechanical axis of the lower limb but internally rotated at 3°.

In this chapter, let us discuss about the etiology, clinical examination, radiological examination, pre-op planning for total knee replacement, intraoperative steps and precautions to take and complications.

2. Valgus deformity in total knee replacement

2.1 Aetiology

Varus or valgus malalignment has a tremendous influence on the loading of the articular surfaces of the knee. This malalignment results in an increased rate of progression of osteoarthrosis in the knee is proven in animal models. The causative factors for valgus deformity of the knee are described as many.

It can be congenital or secondary to osteoarthrosis, rheumatic diseases and post-traumatic arthritis and due to an over-correction consequent to a valgus osteotomy. Valgus deformity in adults is most commonly seen in patients with inflammatory arthritis, tibial malunion, physeal arrest or tibial plateau fracture [2–6]. Persistence of genu valgum from childhood may exist secondary to metabolic disorders, such as rickets and renal osteodystrophy [7]. But in those patients who undergo total knee replacement, osteoarthrosis remains the most common cause.

The pathologic structures which cause the valgus deformity are mainly bony and soft tissue related. Bone factors consist of lateral cartilage erosion, lateral condylar hypoplasia and metaphyseal femur and tibial plateau remodeling. Soft tissue factors include tightening of lateral structures: lateral collateral ligament, posterolateral capsule, popliteus tendon, hamstring tendons, the lateral head of the gastrocnemius and iliotibial band. Rarely, the long head of the biceps femoris is also affected. Lax medial structures (mainly MCL) can add on to the deformity. In addition, these deformities can cause tibial external rotation and to a certain extent patellar lateral subluxation [8]. All these factors in varying severity coexisting around a knee make valgus correction a challenging task during total knee replacement.

2.2 Classifications

Ranawat et al. [9] have described three grades of valgus deformity.

Grade I is where the deformity is less than 10° and it is not a fixed deformity. In Grade I the medial collateral ligament is intact; hence the deformity is passively correctable.

Grade II is featured by a range of deformity from 10 to 20°, whereas the MCL is stretched out but still functional.

Grade III patients have deformity more than 20°. The medial stabilizers are typically not functional, and hence it calls for a constrained implant [9, 10].

Since Ranawat's classification did not take into consideration the extra-articular and multiplanar deformities, Mullaji and Shetty [11] modified it into six types:

Type I—Correctible valgus and an intact MCL.

Type II—Fixed valgus deformity with an intact MCL.

Type III—Valgus and hyperextension deformity with an intact MCL.

Type IV—Valgus and fixed flexion deformity (FFD) with an intact MCL.

Type V—Severe valgus with a lax MCL.

Type VI—Valgus secondary to extra-articular deformity.

Another recently introduced classification system based on the bone affected and the soft tissue status is by the International Society for Technology in Arthroplasty. The JST Classification [12] of valgus knees is as follows:

2.2.1 Femoral deformity

Type F1—Valgus in extension only

- F1a—Intra-articular deformity, loose LCL
- F1b—Extra-articular deformity, normal LCL

Type F2—Valgus in both flexion and extension: Intra-articular deformity, tight lateral collateral ligament, lateral femoral condyle hypoplasia

2.2.2 Tibial deformity

Type T1—Intra-articular deformity, lateral tibial plateau deficiency

Type 2—Extra-articular deformity, tibial metaphyseal or shaft

2.3 Clinical examination

From the history, the most important part is the functional disability the patient is facing and the severity of the pain. Pain, limitation of daily living activities, increasing angular deformity and worsening instability are the usual complaints. The treatment is based on the severity of the symptoms. The co-existence of other pathologies affecting joints like rheumatoid arthritis (RA) and gout has to be evaluated and treated simultaneously.

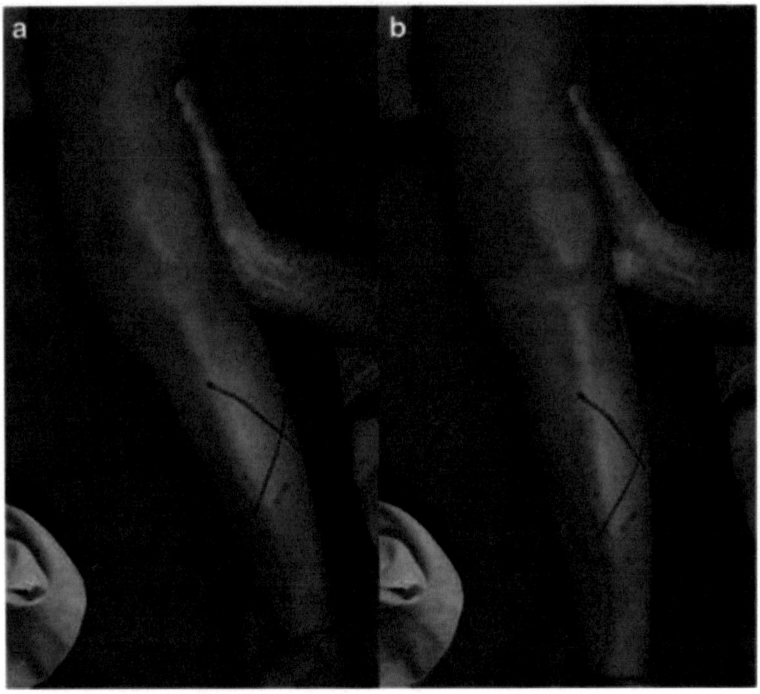

Figure 2.
The valgus deformity corrected with a varus stress test.

First and foremost observation while examining an end-stage degenerative knee disease is the pattern of gait. This is the best way to assess the dynamic instabilities. Due importance should be given if there is a medial thrust and recurvatum/fixed flexion deformity, the amount of deformity and its correctability. **Figure 2** shows the valgus deformity correctability in a varus stress test. The overall alignment should be assessed both in standing and supine positions. The range of motion (ROM) should be measured and recorded. The stability of the knee, anteroposterior laxity, range of motion, coronal and sagittal deformity, mediolateral instability, status of the extensor mechanism and patellofemoral articulation are important in the knee examination.

Lastly, pain due to other causes like neurovascular and lumbosacral pathologies is also to be ruled out. In fixed valgus deformity, the lateral structures are tight, and the medial ligaments are lax. So, when a standard lateral soft tissue release is done, the resulting laxity will be much more than the preoperative, and it usually requires the usage of constrained prosthesis.

2.4 Radiological assessment

A proper radiological evaluation for a valgus knee undergoing TKR includes weight-bearing anteroposterior, lateral, long leg standing, Rosenberg and Merchant views. Lateral views help you size the components and look for any posterior osteophytes. In case of correctable deformities, varus and valgus stress views are mandatory. The critical points to look for in these cases are the amount of bone stock, lateral distal femoral hypoplasia, posterior femoral condyle erosion, metaphyseal remodeling of proximal tibia and distal femur and the status of patella-femoral joint. Patella can be subluxed in case of severe valgus deformities. The depth of resection needs to be planned preoperatively. **Figure 3** shows a valgus knee with lateral tibial

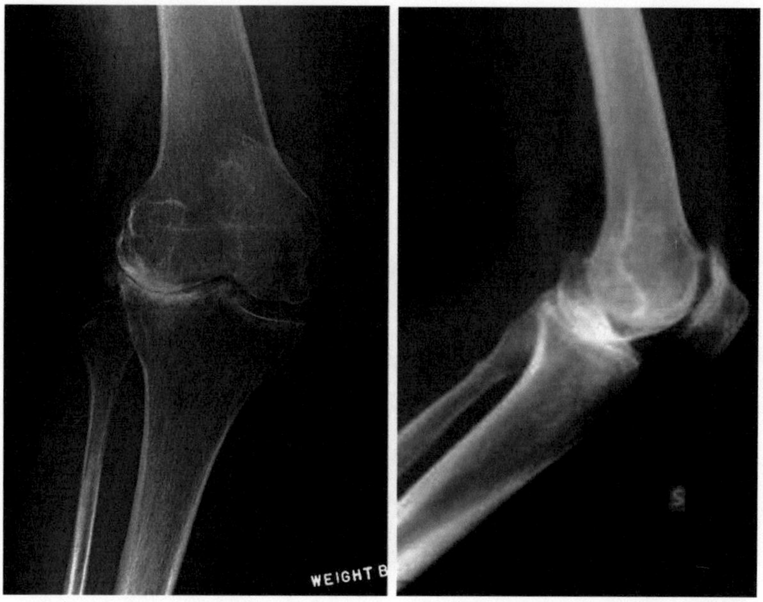

Figure 3.
A valgus knee with lateral tibial plateau defect.

plateau defect. If suspecting bony erosion, a CT scan can help you assess the dimensions of the defect more accurately in order to help you plan the augments early and back it up. Also the hypoplastic lateral femoral condyle, the eroded posterior femoral condyle and the remodeled femoral or tibial metaphysis which can lead to malalignment of the femoral component can be evaluated preoperatively in a CT scan.

Apart from evaluating the knee, plain X-rays of the lumbosacral spine would be worthwhile as a part of ruling out any spine pathology. NCV and EMG may be advised to patients who complain of associated paraesthesia and other sensory or motor symptoms.

2.5 Templating

With the X-rays available, preliminary templating should be done to have a rough idea on the level of resection, valgus angle to keep and sizing of the components. Twenty percent magnification is what most of the templates are made for. Most of the implant companies provide hard copies of TKR templates, or digital templating systems are available.

For the tibia, a line is drawn along tibial anatomical axis, and then a perpendicular one is drawn at the level of the lateral tibial plateau. This will provide the depth of resection to be taken. Try to avoid overhanging. Tibial slope needs to be assessed in lateral view. Some tibial jig/inserts have inbuilt slope. So, thorough knowledge of the system you use is a must to reconstruct the slope.

For measuring the valgus cut angle, the femoral anatomical axis is drawn, and then a second line is drawn from the centre of the intercondylar notch to the centre of the femoral head. The angle formed gives the desired amount of valgus cut to be taken [13] (**Figure 4**).

The sizing of the components is then conducted with the templates provided by the implant company. The femur is sized in lateral view and tibia in AP view. Try to avoid notching in the femur and overhanging in the tibia (**Figure 5**).

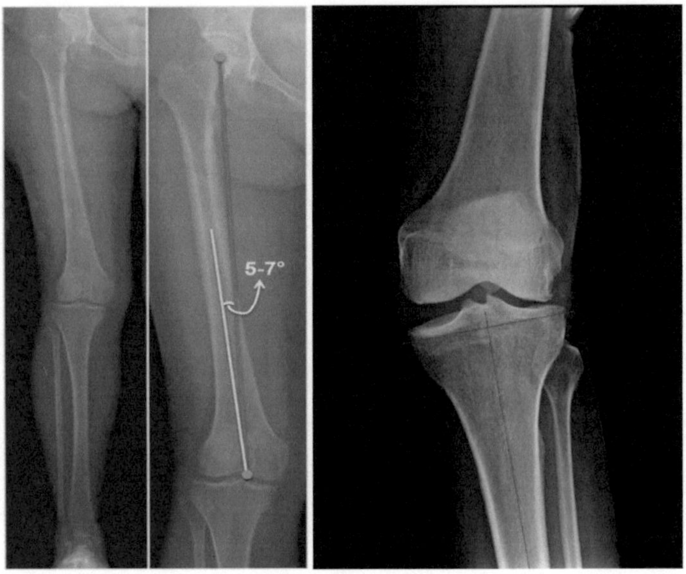

Figure 4.
Templating the bone cuts.

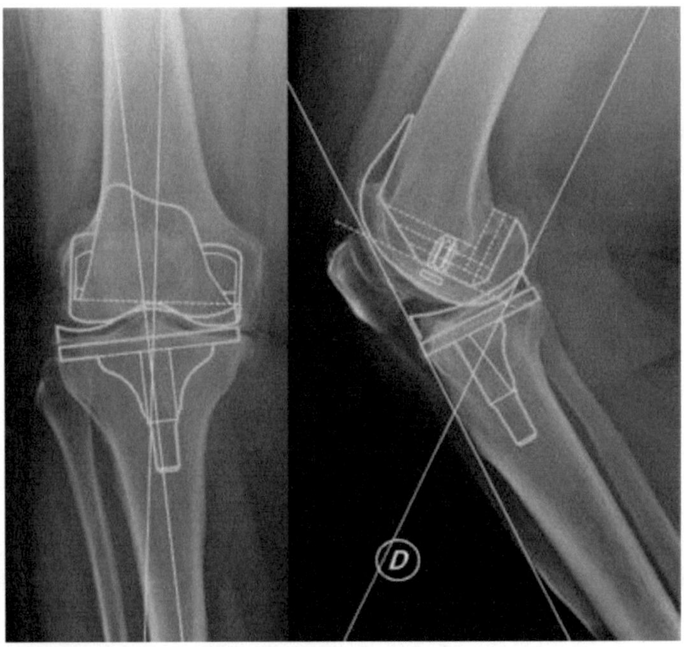

Figure 5.
The digital templates for sizing the components.

2.6 Component selection

Component selection should be made based on the clinical evaluation and the radiological examination. Adequate armamentarium should be ready in the operation theatre (OT) including constrained knee/hinge knee based on the severity of the deformity and its correctability. The final decision is made after bone cuts and soft tissue balancing. If proper soft tissue balance is restored, one can get away with normal components. In a Grade-III valgus deformity, medial soft tissues are not functional, and hence, a higher constrained prosthesis is mandatory to achieve a stable knee [9].

One of the main controversies is regarding the choice and design of the implant to be used in valgus deformities. There are proponents of both the cruciate retaining (CR) and posterior stabilized (PS) designs in existing literature, and they have their valid reasons too. I tend to lean towards PS designs in valgus deformities. PCL is a secondary stabilizer and it is often found contracted intraoperatively [14]. This can limit the deformity correction and almost always end up in resecting PCL too. PS designs are found more stable because of the post-cam mechanism. Also, PS designs allow better lateralization of the components which in turn improve patella tracking. PS prosthesis provides some degree of posterior stabilization as well as protection against posteromedial and posterolateral translation. But the mediolateral laxity is not supported by the PS designs.

Extreme valgus knees will have a deficient lateral femoral condyle. Such knees will require the use of component augmentation if the femoral component is being cemented. The lateral femoral condyle may or may not have distal femoral bone resected like in the chamfer and posterior cuts, as well.

2.7 Intraoperative considerations

The dictum in such complex cases is "plan your work, work out your plan". The plan starts right from the clinical examination. We need to assess whether the valgus deformity is fixed or correctable and the presence of a coexisting deformity—mostly hyperextension. Lateral release should be minimal in case of a fixed deformity because that can make the knee unstable necessitating a constrained prosthesis.

2.7.1 Approach

The knee can be approached both anteromedial and anterolateral. Too much of debate exists on the choice of approach in extreme valgus knees and is often chosen based on the surgeon's preference. The advantages of anterolateral approach as explained by Keblish [8] are better visualization of the tight lateral tissues; lateral release happened with the arthrotomy. Also, if a lateral retinaculum release is necessary, the patellar vascularization will not be compromised. Functional and radiological outcomes in TKA approached either ways have been studied by Sekiya et al. [15]. They found no significant differences in ROM but better postoperative flexion in the anterolateral group. The author is of the opinion that if the residual surgical valgus is more than 15°, it is easier to correct with an anterolateral approach.

2.7.2 Bone cuts

Femur—It is useful to reduce valgus degrees of resection from 5 to 7° to 3° in order to accommodate the distal femoral metaphyseal remodeling. Lateral condyle distal femoral resection can be minimal (1–2 mm) or absent in severe valgus deformity. Femoral resection should be no more than 10 mm in the medial condyle (usually 7–8 mm). Special attention is to be given to lateral condylar hypoplasia that can determine the rotation of the components if a posterior reference is used. In cases of severe trochlear dysplasia, the Whiteside line can be extremely difficult to identify: in these cases the epicondylar axis or parallel to the tibial cut technique should be used to assess a correct femoral rotation.

Tibia—The tibial cut has to be perpendicular to the tibial long axis. The depth of resection should be limited to 6–8 mm in the medial compartment. In cases of severe bony deformity of the tibial plateau, almost no bone is resected on the lateral side to avoid medial over-resection or malaligned cuts.

2.7.3 Soft tissue release

The lateral structures are contracted in valgus knees, and the most important ones to be considered in deformity correction are iliotibial band, posterolateral corner, posterior cruciate ligament, lateral collateral Ligament, popliteus tendon and lateral head of gastrocnemius.

Again controversy exists regarding the sequence and extent of lateral release. Krackow et al. [10] suggest ITB-LCL-popliteus-PLC sequence, whereas Ranawat [9] on the other hand advocates PCL-ITB-LCL technique. Krackow and Mihalko [16] published a cadaveric study in which they studied the amount of correction achieved with each release step of two different sequences, comparing it in flexion and extension. They concluded that LCL release caused largest correction and popliteus, and ITB should be considered to grade the release.

Regarding the technique of release, most of the surgeons do a subperiosteal release from the tibia. In severe valgus deformities, performing a lateral parapatellar approach automatically releases ITB from Gerdy's tubercle and helps in deformity correction to an extent. Ranawat's pie-crusting technique is also done widely. With the knee in extension and lamina spreaders to open up the extension gap, the tight lateral structures are palpated and released by multiple stab incisions with a No. 15 blade (**Figure 6**).

Lateral epicondylar osteotomy as described by Brilhault et al. [17] can be useful in severe valgus deformities. A sliding osteotomy along with the femoral insertion of LCL and popliteus insertions is made, and the bone block is mobilized distally and fixed with screws.

In case of severe valgus deformity, if MCL is attenuated, division and imbrications can be done to tighten the medial structures. Other options are distalizing the PLC insertion from the tibia and fixation with trans-osseous sutures. In all those cases requiring such measures, a constrained condylar prosthesis is the norm.

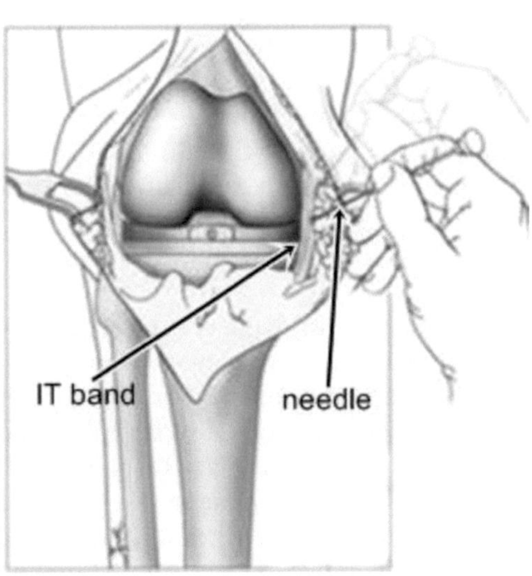

Figure 6.
Ranawat's pie-crusting technique for extensive lateral release

Based on JST Classification of valgus knees, an intraoperative algorithm is given below [12].

2.7.3.1 Type F1a

Deformity is due to tight ITB and posterior-lateral capsule instead of LCL and popliteus tendon. Releasing ITB and posterior-lateral capsule can correct the deformity. Additionally, a bony graft or a metal block may be used to augment the hypoplastic lateral distal femoral condyle.

2.7.3.2 Type F1b

Deformity is at the level of supra-condylar region. Three options are used based on the severity of deformity.

Option 1—Lateral condyle distal sliding osteotomy is done to convert an F1b deformity into an F1a deformity. The procedure brings the deformity level into the collateral ligament level.

Option 2—Soft tissue release + constrained prosthesis.

Option 3—One-stage or two-stage supra-condylar osteotomy + TKA.

F1b valgus knee is due to supra-condylar deformity; a supra-condylar osteotomy (SCO) can aid in balancing. SCO + TKA can be done in a single stage, but be careful about the cortical break while inserting the IM rod. Also femoral stem extension may be needed in such cases; hence there can be a serious compromise in the blood supply to the osteotomy site causing non-union.

2.7.3.3 Type F2

Both the distal and posterior parts of LFC are deficient; LCL is contracted. The release of lateral soft tissues, including LCL and popliteus, may become essential.

2.7.3.4 Type T deformity

This is rare and mostly seen in rheumatoids or post-traumatic cases. The reconstruction of the plateau can be done with augments in T1 knee, and corrective osteotomy may be required for a T2 knee.

2.8 My preferred technique

Approach—Medial parapatellar approach. Careful not to release medial structures much, minimizing medial dissection to fully expose the tibia. If under anesthesia valgus correction is more than 15°; lateral parapatellar approach is preferred.

Implant—PS only. It is important to keep the condylar knee constrained and rotate the hinge knee as back up based on the severity and pathology of valgus.

Femur first—Reduce the valgus degree of resection to 3°; the entry point for IM rod in a valgus knee is usually more medial than in a standard knee. Ascertain the point with preoperative radiographs. With regard to anteroposterior cuts, watch out for hypoplasia of the lateral femoral condyle, and check the posterior condylar reference cutting block position with both Whiteside line and transepicondylar axis. Also, with the cutting blocks fixed, further check the balancing in flexion before performing the cuts.

Perform the tibial cut, perpendicular to the anatomical axis, allowing 3–5° posterior slope using an extramedullary rod. Try to remove the least possible bone amount, especially from the lateral side.

Extension gap is assessed using lamina spreaders and limited lateral release—pie crusting or ITB release is done to make it rectangular. Popliteus has to be preserved as it is a stabilizer in flexion. Varus-valgus stability is assessed in extension. Once the knee is balanced in extension, the flexion gap can be evaluated and assessed. When the knee is balanced, femoral chamfer cuts are made, and the trial components can be tested.

With trial femur, tibia and insert, it is important to assess patella tracking. If needed, a lateral retinacular release can be done inside out at this stage.

2.9 Complications

Complications which can happen in correcting a valgus deformity in TKR include tibiofemoral instability, residual valgus deformity (most common ones), restricted ROM, wound dehiscence, patella fracture, patella maltracking and peroneal nerve palsy. Correction of a severe valgus deformity can induce peroneal nerve injury due to traction or ischemia.

So, it is of utmost importance to specifically mention these complications to the patient and bystanders and get a well-informed consent prior to surgery.

2.10 Clinical outcomes

Revision rates following TKA for valgus knees at 10–15-year follow-up have been reported at between 0 and 17% [18]. Failure rate is more when the preoperative deformity is more or the residual valgus is more. The long-term results of TKA in valgus knees are reported to be not up to that of varus knees.

3. Conclusion

Valgus deformity correction in total knee replacement is not everyone's cup of coffee. Associated bone defects and ligamentous contractures add to the difficulty. Sequential release of the lateral tight structures, correcting the deformity and balancing the knee, is a tricky job. A thorough planning, surgical skill, adequate implant back up and an active physiotherapy team are mandatory to achieve the desired functional results in a valgus knee TKR.

Conflict of interest

There is no conflict of interest to declare.

Author details

Melvin J. George
Sree Narayana Institute of Medical Sciences, Kochi, Kerala, India

*Address all correspondence to: johnirimpenz@yahoo.co.in

References

[1] Paley D, Tetsworth K. Mechanical axis deviation of the lower limbs. Preoperative planning of uniapical angular deformities of the tibia or femur. Clinical Orthopaedics and Related Research. 1992 Jul;**280**:48-64

[2] Favorito PJ, Mihalko WM, Krackow KA. Total knee arthroplasty in the valgus knee. The Journal of the American Academy of Orthopaedic Surgeons. 2002;**10**(1):16-24

[3] Rossi R, Rosso F, Cottino U, Dettoni F, Bonasia DE, Bruzzone M. Total knee arthroplasty in the valgus knee. International Orthopaedics. 2014;**38**:273-283

[4] Apostolopoulos AP, Nikolopoulos DD, Polyzois I, Nakos A, Liarokapis S, Stefanakis G, et al. Total knee arthroplasty in severe valgus deformity: Interest of combining a lateral approach with a tibial tubercle osteotomy. Orthopaedics & Traumatology, Surgery & Research. 2010;**96**:777-784

[5] Nikolopoulos DD, Polyzois I, Apostolopoulos AP, Rossas C, Moutsios-Rentzos A, Michos IV. Total knee arthroplasty in severe valgus knee deformity: Comparison of a standard medial parapatellar approach combined with tibial tubercle osteotomy. Knee Surgery, Sports Traumatology, Arthroscopy. 2011;**19**:1834-1842

[6] Karachalios T, Sarangi PP, Newman JH. Severe varus and valgus deformities treated by total knee arthroplasty. Journal of Bone and Joint Surgery. British Volume (London). 1994;**76**:938-942

[7] White GR, Mencio GA. Genu Valgum in children: Diagnostic and therapeutic alternatives. The Journal of the American Academy of Orthopaedic Surgeons. 1995;**3**:275-283

[8] Keblish PA. The lateral approach to the valgus knee. Surgical technique and analysis of 53 cases with over two-year follow-up evaluation. Clinical Orthopaedics and Related Research. 1991;**271**:52-62

[9] Ranawat AS, Ranawat CS, Elkus M, Rasquinha VJ, Rossi R, Babhulkar S. Total knee arthroplasty for severe valgus deformity. The Journal of Bone and Joint Surgery. American Volume. 2005;**87**(Suppl 1):271-284

[10] Krackow KA, Jones MM, Teeny SM, Hungerford DS. Primary total knee arthroplasty in patients with fixed valgus deformity. Clinical Orthopaedics and Related Research. 1991;**273**:9-18

[11] Mullaji AB, Shetty GM. Deformity Correction in Total Knee Arthroplasty. New York: Springer Science and Business Media; 2014. pp. 59-71

[12] Zhou Y. JST classification and treatment algorithm of a valgus knee. Orthopaedic Proceedings;**92-B** (Suppl 1). International Society for Technology in Arthroplasty. 2018

[13] Nogueira JBS, do Carmo Araújo LH, Bezerra MJC. Planning Total Knee Arthroplasties. Croatia, Rijeka: Intech Open Publishers; 2018

[14] Krackow KA. The Technique of Total Knee Arthroplasty. Mosby, St. Louis; 1990

[15] Sekiya H, Takatoku K, Takada H, Sugimoto N, Hoshino Y. Lateral approach is advantageous in total knee arthroplasty for valgus deformed knee. European Journal of Orthopaedic Surgery and Traumatology. 2014 Jan;**24**(1):111-115

[16] Krackow KA, Mihalko WM. Flexion-extension joint gap changes after lateral structure release for

valgus deformity correction in total knee arthroplasty: A cadaveric study. The Journal of Arthroplasty. 1999;**14**(8):994-1004

[17] Brilhault J, Lautman S, Favard L, Burdin P. Lateral femoral sliding osteotomy lateral release in total knee arthroplasty for a fixed valgus deformity. Journal of Bone and Joint Surgery. British Volume (London). 2002;**84**(8):1131-1137

[18] Elkus M, Ranawat CS, Rasquinha VJ, et al. Total knee arthroplasty for severe valgus deformity. Five to fourteen-year follow-up. Journal of Bone and Joint Surgery 2004;**86-A**:2671-2676